Narrative Medicine

THE FIFTH VITAL SIGN

ARTHUR LAZARUS, MD, MBA

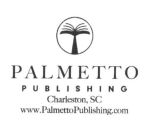

PALMETTO
P U B L I S H I N G
Charleston, SC
www.PalmettoPublishing.com

Paperback ISBN: 979-8-8229-3898-4
eBook ISBN: 979-8-8229-3899-1

ALSO BY ARTHUR LAZARUS

Neuroleptic Malignant Syndrome and Related Conditions (co-author)

Controversies in Managed Mental Health Care

Career Pathways in Psychiatry: Transition in Changing Times

*MD/MBA: Physicians on the New Frontier of
Medical Management*

*Every Story Counts: Examining Contemporary Practice Through
Narrative Medicine*

Medicine on Fire: A Narrative Travelogue

"This is the basic human story. We are all on the same journey. Every one of us will suffer – there's no way around it. The crucial question is not how to avoid suffering, it's how we move through it."
— Samuel Shem, *The House of God*

Contents

About the Author

Arthur L. Lazarus, MD, MBA, is a healthcare consultant, certified physician executive, and nationally recognized author, speaker, and champion of physician leadership and wellness. He has broad experience in clinical practice and the health insurance industry, having led programs at Cigna and Humana. At Humana, Lazarus was vice president and corporate medical director of behavioral health operations in Louisville, Kentucky, and subsequently a population health medical director for the state of Florida.

Lazarus has also held leadership positions in several pharmaceutical companies, including Pfizer and AstraZeneca, conducting clinical trials, and reviewing promotional material for medical accuracy and FDA compliance. He has published more than 250 articles in scientific and professional journals and has written six books, including *Neuroleptic Malignant Syndrome and Related Conditions, Controversies in Managed Mental Health Care, Career Pathways in Psychiatry, MD/MBA: Physicians on the New Frontier of Medical Management, Every Story Counts: Exploring Contemporary Practice Through Narrative Medicine, and Medicine on Fire: A Narrative Travelogue.*

Born in Philadelphia, Pennsylvania, Lazarus attended Boston University, where he graduated with a bachelor's degree in psychology with Distinction. He received his medical degree with Honors from Temple University School of Medicine, followed by a psychiatric residency at Temple University Hospital, where he was chief resident. After residency, Lazarus joined the faculty of Temple University School of Medicine, where he currently serves as adjunct professor of Psychiatry. He also holds non-faculty appointments as Executive-in-Residence at Temple University Fox School of Business and Management, where he received his MBA degree, and Senior Fellow, Jefferson College of Population Health, Philadelphia, Pennsylvania.

Well known for his leadership and medical management skills, Lazarus is a sought-after presenter, mentor, teacher, and writer. He has shared his expertise and perspective at numerous local, national, and international meetings and seminars.

Lazarus is a past president of the American Association for Psychiatric Administration and Leadership, a former member of the board of directors of the American Association for Physician Leadership (AAPL), and a current member of the AAPL editorial review board. In 2010, the American Psychiatric Association honored Lazarus with the Administrative Psychiatry Award for his effectiveness as an administrator of major mental health programs and expanding the body of knowledge of management science in mental health services delivery systems.

Lazarus is among a select group of physicians in the United States who have been inducted into both the Alpha Omega Alpha medical honor society and the Beta Gamma Sigma honor society of collegiate schools of business.

Lazarus lives with his wife near Charlotte, North Carolina. They have four adult children. He enjoys walking, biking, playing piano, and listening to music.

Preface

Chris Adrian begins his "Grand Rounds" talk as follows: "'Narrative Medicine.' What does that even mean? 'Narrative Medicine.' I'm never totally sure what that means, but I think that's part of the point, that it means different things to different people, and that, just because the phrase 'Narrative Medicine' contains the word 'medicine' you can't expect it to mean the same thing to everyone…"

Adrian is a renowned physician author and pediatric hematologist/oncologist at Columbia University. Columbia is considered the birthplace of narrative medicine. The "movement" was started by Rita Charon, MD, PhD, and codified in her 2006 textbook *Narrative Medicine: Honoring the Stories of Illness*, essentially a call to action for doctors "to honor the meanings of their patients' narratives of illness, and to be moved by what they behold so that they can act on their patients' behalf." What Charon and her colleagues termed "narrative medicine" was further defined as "medicine practiced with the narrative competence to recognize, absorb, interpret, and be moved by the stories of illness."

Charon also supplied the answer to the frequently asked question: why study and teach narrative medicine? She wrote: "Narrative medicine makes the case that narrative training in reading and writing contributes to clinical effectiveness. By developing narrative competence, we have argued, health care professionals can become more attentive to patients, more attuned to patients' experiences, more reflective in their own practice, and more accurate in interpreting the stories patients tell of illness."

Both Charon and Adrian are correct in that narrative medicine must be experienced, and it can be difficult to characterize unless one has practiced medicine or has been a patient. Although the field is still evolving, it remains an indispensable resource for understanding the individual, patient-specific meaning of an illness and a doctor's reaction to it.

There are many different perspectives and philosophies of narrative medicine. At least four genres can be distinguished: (1) **Patient Stories** – classic illness narratives written by patients; (2) **Physicians' Stories**, often laced with memoir; (3) **Narratives about Physician-Patient Encounters**; and (4) **Grand Stories**, so-called "metanarratives" of sociocultural understandings of the body in health and illness.

I gravitate quite naturally toward writing narratives detailing "physician stories." But I also like to teach, so, for this book, my third collection of essays, I decided to include some that are instructional – a primer if you will – to give writing tips to students of all ages and to outline some basic writing rules and tools we should respect. The final product is one-third instruction (Section 1) and two-thirds inspiration (Section 2).

Most of the essays were written during the fall and winter of 2023. I was enrolled in a narrative healthcare course at a local university. It might sound cliché, but the most important lessons I learned were: (1) do not be afraid to write; (2) do not fear being criticized; and (3) write using the strength of your inner voice.

I don't worry that my prose can't compete with Abraham Verghese's, that my narratives may not be as spiritual as Lewis Mehl-Madrona's, that my storytelling isn't as unconventional Amy Hempel's, or that my memoirs are not as deeply rooted as Patricia Hampl's. No one's are.

What you *will find* between the covers of this book – to quote Hampl – is "the intersection of narration and reflection, of storytelling and essay writing," draped in a style of narrative medicine I call all my own.

May you find your way as pleasant.

To my mentors and mentees, in appreciation.

INSTRUCTION

1.
Kick Start Your Writing with a Surprise

Our life's journey is not always apparent, and neither is our written destination.

One of the most memorable scenes in Goodfellas occurs early on, when the audience is introduced to most of the crew at the Bamboo Lounge. Henry Hill (Ray Liotta) and Tommy DeVito (Joe Pesci) get into a tense exchange. Tommy seems to become offended after Henry calls him funny. "I'm funny how, Tommy wants to know?" "I mean, funny like a clown? I amuse you? I make you laugh?"

Unknown to the other actors, the scene was being improvised, although it was based on a true incident. A young Pesci was a waiter at a restaurant and told a mobster that he was funny. Needless to say, the wise guy didn't take this compliment too well. Director Martin Scorsese wanted the dialog between Pesci and Liotta to be improvised because he wanted to capture the unrehearsed reactions of the actors.

Clearly, that is one way to make a story impactful: through improvisation and authentic dialog, i.e., dialogue used to reveal character traits and advance the story. The fun in writing, many people say, is surprising yourself as you write. You begin with an idea and simply start typing, not knowing exactly where you are going. You pause to reflect or daydream, and suddenly a memory or old lesson pops into your head. This moment of surprising yourself with your own thoughts can translate into words on a blank canvas, and it is at the heart of good writing and even songwriting.

Paul Simon said he trusted his spontaneity when he wrote "You Can Call Me Al." Simon remarked: "I'm more interested in what I discover than what I invent." Elaborating on the distinction between discovery and invention, Simon continued, "You just have no idea that that's a thought that you had; it surprises you; it can make me laugh or make me emotional. When it happens and I'm the audience and I react, I have faith in that because I'm already reacting. I don't have to question it. I've already been the audience. But if I make it up, knowing where it's going, it's not as much fun. It may be just as good, but it's more fun to discover it."

The title of Simon's eleventh studio solo album is, in fact, "Surprise," and it features a baby's face on the cover to illustrate the sense of wonder and new discovery found within songwriting and writing in general. Children surprise us all the time with their imagination and insight, challenging our own fixed assumptions and perceptions. In *Poetic Medicine*, certified poetry therapist John Fox observed: "The statement 'I had no idea my child thought that way' is exactly what many adults wanted to hear from their own parents but didn't." If you're someone who "didn't hear it" from your parents, it's not too late to unearth your creativity and incorporate the element of surprise in your writing, especially in health narratives, as you discover your true voice.

We often think of "surprise" as a powerful tool to engage readers, keeping them interested, and making the narrative more memorable. But writing health narratives can be a surprising process for the writers themselves due to several reasons:

1. **Unforeseen insights.** While writing, physicians may discover new insights about a situation, condition, or patient that they hadn't realized before. This could be a different perspective, a deeper understanding of a

medical condition, or a newfound appreciation for a particular treatment approach.

2. **Emotional discoveries.** Health narratives often involve delving into deep emotional territories. As physicians explore these areas, they might surprise themselves with the depth of their own emotional responses, empathy, or resilience. Writing health narratives has been shown to help clinicians better appreciate the importance of the emotion and intersubjective relation borne of the telling of and listening to patients' stories.

3. **Unplanned directions.** Sometimes, a narrative can take an unexpected turn as it develops. A physician might start with an idea or a plan, but as they delve deeper into the narrative, they find it evolving in ways they didn't initially anticipate. My creative writing instructor told our class that narrative medicine writing "opens the conversation to magic," meaning the creative direction and nature of the narrative can be limitless. Lewis Mehl-Madrona, MD, PhD, a name synonymous with the narrative medicine movement, observed that physicians may see themselves "as coauthors in the creation of new stories that have uncertain endings, at least while they are being written."

4. **Self-reflection.** Writing health narratives can lead to significant self-reflection. Physicians may surprise themselves by uncovering personal biases, strengths, weaknesses, or beliefs that they weren't previously aware of. Narrative medicine reflective writing has been used to help promote incorporation of diversity, equity, and inclusion training into medical school curricula.

5. **New connections.** As clinicians delve into the intricacies of health narratives, they might discover surprising connections between disparate ideas, events, or facts. These connections can add depth and complexity to the narrative.

6. **Therapeutic impact.** Many physicians find the process of writing health narratives to be therapeutic. The act of writing can help them process their experiences, emotions, and thoughts, leading to surprising personal revelations or growth. Some physicians' careers have been totally revitalized by writing real-life stories about the joys and challenges of practicing medicine in the modern era.

7. **Enhanced skills.** Through the process of writing and revising, physicians often surprise themselves with the improvement in their writing skills, ability to articulate complex ideas, and capacity to engage readers in a meaningful way. Adopting narrative medicine as an intervention in medical education has played an important role in the professional identity development of medical students.

8. **Patient outcomes.** Writing about patients' stories might lead to surprising revelations about patients' resilience, their responses to treatment, or their coping mechanisms, which can add a new layer of understanding to the narrative.

The element of surprise certainly factored into this essay. I had originally planned to write about rules for writing health narratives, such as "show, don't tell," first do background research, and so on (see the next essay). I sat down with that blank canvas, began typing, and my 3-year-old grandson barged into the office and exclaimed, "Bops, man, how 'ya doin'?" ("Bops" is a neologism for "Pops" and "Bebop." He knows I love music.) His surprise attack, coupled with my thinking about the beauty and innocence of children, steered me in a different direction – that is, toward writing this essay.

"Kids do say the darndest things," Art Linkletter used to say. Whenever I get stuck at writing, I begin to think like a child to spur myself on. "It takes a long time to become young," noted Pablo Picasso.

2.
A Few Rules to Consider When Writing Narratives

Number 1: You rule!

Although I rarely eat at Outback Steakhouse, I've admired the Australian-themed restaurant chain's longstanding motto: "No Rules." Deep down, I dislike rules. A psychologist told me he could tell I was "anti-authoritarian" – without formally testing me. A psychiatrist described me as irreverent. They were both correct. Essentially, I do not follow the rules (just ask my wife!).

The fact that there are very few writing rules in narrative medicine is one of the features that attracts me to it. But that doesn't mean you can write willy-nilly. What you put on paper begins with an understanding of the context of the narrative, and it must encompass several other attributes.

The **context** of a narrative is more than just background information. It is a vital part of understanding and treating the patient effectively. Clearly, the context of a narrative is crucial because it sets the stage for understanding the story, event, or situation being described. In a clinical setting, the context may include patient history, current symptoms, recent changes, and environmental factors. It provides necessary information that helps physicians and other healthcare providers interpret the patient's condition accurately. Setting the proper context for your narrative is key to making it impactful.

Authentic dialog, i.e., dialog used to reveal character traits and advance the story, is equally important. The characters are real people, usually patients, and they should be portrayed with depth and complexity. This includes showing their motivations, conflicts, growth, and changes over time. The dialog must therefore be authentic and reflective of the character's personality, background, and time period.

Truth and accuracy are paramount in medical narratives. The events, characters, dialogues, and settings must be as accurate as possible. Narrative medicine is a form of creative nonfiction. That means your narratives can (and should) be creative, but they can't take liberties with the truth. Often the "truth" must be reconstructed from memory, which could introduce historical distortion into the narrative. That's understood and considered okay in the world of narrative medicine, especially memoir, as long as the accounts actually occurred and are retold to the best of your ability.

While maintaining factual accuracy, writers can use **literary devices** such as foreshadowing, flashback, symbolism, metaphor, and simile to enhance the narrative. These literary devices can help physicians gain a deeper understanding of a patient's perspective. They can also make the narrative more engaging and memorable, thus improving communication and empathy between healthcare providers and patients.

Show, don't tell, is probably the closest thing to a commandment in narrative medicine writing. You should aim to create vivid imagery and provoke emotion through detailed descriptions and accounts, rather than simply stating facts. Some authors suggest that you should show *and* tell. You are creating a work of art, not writing a patient's progress note or legal document.

Your narrative can be **structured** in various ways; it doesn't have to follow a linear timeline. However, the structure should serve the story and make it engaging for the reader. Because writing narratives often involves your reflection on the events – thoughts, feelings, and learning from the experience – a well-structured narrative allows for more effective **reflection**, as it provides a clear, organized account of the patient's experiences. Structure and reflection are two critical components that work together: structure provides the necessary framework for the narrative, while reflection allows for the extraction of meaningful insights from the story, leading to a more empathetic and comprehensive understanding of the patient's condition and experience.

Since narrative medicine is based on real events and people, thorough **research** is essential. This can include interviews, reading documents or reports, visiting locations, etc. Good old-fashioned literature reviews are not out of the question, either. PubMed, a free web-based interface for searching MEDLINE, has been essential in my quest for scholarly knowledge that I integrate into narratives. PubMed has information about journal articles (approximately 25 million) published in 5,600 journals in 30 languages dating back to 1946. I probably spend as much or more time researching a topic as I do writing about it.

You should respect the **privacy and dignity** of the people you write about. This might involve changing names or identifying details, particularly in sensitive situations. Asking patients and families for permission to share their stories is never a bad idea. Maintaining compliance with HIPAA is always a must. The physician and poet William Carlos Williams (1883-1963) wrote: "Their story, yours, mine – it's what we carry with us on this trip we take, and we owe it to each other to **respect our stories** (bold font added) and learn from them."

As with all writing, **revision** is key in narrative medicine. This involves reviewing your work for clarity, coherence, grammar, punctuation, and overall flow (see essay 13). Don't become overly obsessive, but check your work a few times before you consider it final. And don't get hung up on precise phraseology. Recreations of the past can change (see "truth" above). Be satisfied with your completed narrative, recognizing that it has inherent limitations owing to its inevitable subjectivity and point of view. There are many ways to say the same thing and convey the same meaning, and next time you may choose to do it differently.

Remember, while these are general rules, narrative medicine is a flexible genre and allows for considerable experimentation. Ultimately, there is only one rule to follow: You tell me your story; I'll tell you mine.

3.
What Qualities do Psychiatrists Possess that Prepare Them for Storytelling and Narrative Medicine Writing?

"Psychiatry is the art of teaching people how to stand on their own feet while reclining on couches."
– Sigmund Freud

Psychiatric training prepares physicians to be a good managers. There are many parallels between the roles of therapists and administrators, such as (1) tolerance of ambiguity, (2) complex decision-making abilities, (3) appropriate use of judgment to solve people's problems, (4) counseling upset and angry people, (5) introducing change and overcoming resistance to change, and (6) managing time and finances.

I wondered whether a similar parallel existed with respect to narrative medicine. In other words, can psychiatric training help someone become a better storyteller and medical writer? And if so, how? I had to think long and hard about this question. While combing the medical literature, I found no precedent for answering it. Actually, quite the opposite, I came across an article titled: "The Value and Benefit of Narrative Medicine for Psychiatric Practice." The article described how literary studies were able to help the author understand and formulate psychiatric histories, but not necessarily how to write better assessments.

While reflecting on my experience as a psychiatrist, I was able to uncover certain qualities in my training and practice that might have aided me in writing narratives:

1. **Empathy**: Psychiatry is a field that involves a deep understanding of patients' emotions and experiences. This empathy can translate into powerful storytelling as psychiatrists can put themselves into their patients' shoes and narrate their experiences with sensitivity and accuracy.

2. **Observation**: Psychiatrists spend a lot of time observing their patients, noting changes in behavior, speech, and emotions. This keen sense of observation can lend itself well to descriptive writing, as they can detail situations and characters in a way that brings the story to life.

3. **Understanding of Human Psychology**: Psychiatrists have a profound understanding of human psychology; some, like myself, majored in psychology in college. However, approximately half of psychiatrists nowadays do not incorporate psychotherapy in their practice. Nevertheless, psychiatrists are trained to understand why people behave the way they do, what motivates them, and how they react in different situations. This knowledge can add depth and complexity to their characters and narratives.

4. **Communication Skills**: Good psychiatrists are adept communicators. They know how to ask the right questions, listen actively, and convey information effectively. These skills can be beneficial in narrative medicine writing where clear, concise communication is key.

5. **Confidentiality**: Psychiatrists are bound by patient-doctor confidentiality, meaning they are trusted with personal and sensitive information.

While they cannot share specific details about their patients, their experience dealing with such information can lend a sense of authenticity and respect to their narratives (see previous essay).

6. **Analytical Skills**: Psychiatrists are trained to analyze symptoms, behaviors, and situations to form a diagnosis. These analytical skills can be useful in storytelling as they can help in developing a plot and understanding character motivations.

7. **Patience**: The nature of psychiatry often requires patience, as progress can be slow and setbacks common. This patience can translate into a thoughtful and careful approach to storytelling, where every detail is considered, every development is thoroughly explained, and the writing process itself can be very slow.

8. **Creativity**: While psychiatry is a science, it also requires creativity, especially when it comes to problem-solving and treatment strategies. This creativity can also be channeled into narrative medicine writing, making for compelling and engaging stories (see essay 37).

9. **Memory**: Practicing psychiatry relies heavily on memory and on the ability to retrieve and organize images and events from the past. Remembering events and their sequence can help in creating a coherent and compelling storyline. Recall aids in the recollection of specific details that can enrich a narrative. It could be colors, smells, sounds, or feelings. These details can make a story more vivid and immersive.

The renowned psychiatrist and psychoanalyst Carl Jung spoke to the transformative nature of human connections, which is often at the heart of storytelling. He said: "The meeting of two personalities is like the contact of two chemical substances: if there is any reaction, both are transformed."

Of course, psychiatric training is not a prerequisite for good writing and storytelling. Harvard-trained physician Michael Crichton is an example.

He felt medical school was valuable not only to his career as a writer and storyteller, but also as a movie director. Crichton commented: "Being a doctor is good preparation for this [directing], because it teaches you to deal with the kind of life that you will inevitably have. It teaches you to work well when you haven't had enough sleep. It teaches you to work well when you're on your feet a lot. It teaches you to work well with technical problems and it teaches you to make decisions and then live by them. I think it also has advantages in working with actors, because one of the things a doctor has to learn is to be able to meet a patient whom he has never seen before and rapidly assess him in terms of what kind of person he is, and not merely whether he's perforated his ulcer. You've got to be able to analyze just what kind of person you're dealing with."

The Russian playwright and short-story writer Anton Chekov is considered to be among the greatest writers of short fiction in history. His writing career predated his medical career. His stories and plays reveal the insights that Chekhov discovered about the human psyche at work, thus delving into psychosomatic medicine nearly 50 years before its time.

There are many other physicians-turned-authors, past and present, too numerous to mention. Some are discussed in essay 6. Perhaps you'll be the next one.

4.
Reading Informs Writing

Every physician knows the tried-and-true method of learning: "see one, do one, teach one." In narrative medicine, we might say: "read many, write many, publish at least one."

They say that reading – close reading – imparts good writing skills. What is close reading? Why is reading important for writing medical narratives? What type of reading is critical to students of the narrative? Let's take a "closer" look at these questions, one at a time.

"Close reading" in narrative medicine refers to the attentive and thorough examination of a text, often a patient's narrative or story. This type of reading goes beyond simply understanding the literal meaning of the words. It involves a deep analysis of the language used, the structure of the narrative, and the context in which it is given. The aim is to gain a deeper understanding of the patient's experience, their perceptions, emotions, and the meanings they attribute to their illness. It can involve analyzing the choice of words, metaphors, and symbols used by the patient, as well as the tone, rhythm, and pace of their speech.

Close reading allows healthcare providers to understand not just the medical facts, but also the personal, social, and emotional dimensions of illness. This can lead to more empathetic, patient-centered care and better therapeutic relationships. It can also provide valuable insights for diagnosis, treatment planning, and patient education.

Close reading is integral to the teaching of narrative medicine at the College of Physicians and Surgeons of Columbia University. Faculty are required to read what their students write, so they must be trained in close reading themselves. Columbia's institution-wide effort to teach close reading and creative writing aims to equip students, residents, and faculty with the prerequisites to provide attentive, empathic clinical care.

Josephine Ensign, author and professor of nursing at the University of Washington, wrote: "I find that it [the close reading drill used at Columbia] is too cold, cerebral, intellectual; to practice it somehow further objectifies the 'patient' and holds them at arm's length in order to dissect and measure." Ensign felt it was necessary to revise the drill for her students. Here is her modified version taught at the University of Washington in Seattle:

- **Emotion**: What do you feel while reading this (or while listening to this patient illness narrative)? What is the overall mood or emotional effect of the piece? And why do you think it evokes this particular response for you?

- **Surprise**: What stands out to you the most? What is unexpected? What distracts you but is not the focus of the narrative?

- **Silence**. What is unsaid in this? Whose voices or perspectives are included and whose are left out?

- **Metaphor** (and its close cousin simile). The use of imagery and the poetics of the piece.

As for the second question, why is reading important for medical narrative writing, I can think of several reasons:

1. **Vocabulary and Language Skills**: Reading a wide variety of materials can help expand your medical and general vocabulary, enhancing your ability to express ideas clearly and precisely.

2. **Understanding Structure**: Reading can help you understand how ideas and information are organized within a text, which can improve your ability to write structured and coherent narratives.

3. **Improving Analytical Skills**: Reading can also improve your ability to analyze and interpret information, which is crucial when writing about complex medical cases.

4. **Developing Empathy**: Reading about diverse experiences can help you develop empathy, which is crucial for writing narratives that accurately and sensitively reflect patients' experiences.

5. **Keeping Updated**: Reading the latest medical literature can help you stay updated on the latest research and developments, which can inform your writing and make it more relevant and accurate.

Reading a variety of materials can greatly enhance the skills needed for writing medical narratives. Here are a few types of reading that could be particularly beneficial:

1. **Medical literature**: Reading medical literature such as research papers, case studies, and articles in medical journals can provide a solid understanding of the language, style, and structure commonly used in medical writing. It can also help to build a broad medical vocabulary and an understanding of how to present complex ideas in a clear, concise manner. Understanding the "language of medicine" is fundamental to being able to write about it.

2. **Clinical guidelines and protocols**: These provide a structured approach to patient care and can help in understanding how to organize and present

information logically and systematically. They also often contain examples of how to document patient interactions, treatment plans, and outcomes.

3. **Medically-oriented literature**: Reading high-quality medically-oriented literature, including novels, newspapers, and magazines, can help to develop a strong command of language and an ability to write in a clear, engaging style. It can also help to build empathy and understanding, which are crucial in writing about patients' experiences and perspectives. A brief list of notable authors and books is presented in essay 6.

4. **Patient narratives**: Reading narratives written by patients can provide insight into the patient perspective, helping to develop compassion and understanding. This can lead to more patient-centered writing, reflecting not just the medical facts but also the human side of medicine, helping healthcare professionals provide more empathetic and effective care. Here are a few examples:

1. *The Diving Bell and the Butterfly* by Jean-Dominique Bauby: This memoir was written by a former editor-in-chief of *French Elle* magazine, who suffered a stroke and became paralyzed with the only exception of some movement in his head and eyes ("locked-in syndrome"). He wrote the entire book by blinking his left eye.

2. *Autobiography of a Face* by Lucy Grealy: This memoir explores the author's experience with Ewing's sarcoma, a cancer that severely disfigured her face.

3. *My Stroke of Insight* by Jill Bolte Taylor: A neuroanatomist's account of her own stroke and recovery provides unique insights into the workings of the brain.

4. *The Cancer Journals* by Audre Lorde: Lorde's account of her breast cancer and mastectomy explores her own feelings about the disease, her treatment, and societal attitudes toward illness and disability.

5. *The Last Lecture* by Randy Pausch: A computer science professor at Carnegie Mellon University, who was diagnosed with terminal cancer, shares his thoughts on living a fulfilling life.

6. *Sickened: The Memoir of a Munchausen by Proxy Childhood* by Julie Gregory: A memoir of a young girl who is forced into being a patient by her mother who suffers from Munchausen syndrome by proxy, a form of child abuse (see essay 33).

5.
How Should a Good Narrative Appear to Readers?

Oops…I forgot to add: creative.

Once in a while I'll publish an essay on Medium (https://medium.com), an Internet blog and online hybrid collection of amateur and professional writers and publications. It's my least preferred option because the website is not medically oriented and it's very crowded with lots of submissions competing to be read. I think the most successful articles on Medium – the ones that attract the most readers – are the articles that have the broadest appeal by virtue of their titles. Here are some examples (there's no accounting for taste):

- Top 20 Mobile Apps Which Nobody Knows About

- How to Identify a Narcissist

- Hello, I Have Amazing Boobs

- The Email that Ended My 20 Year Marriage

- At 68, I'm Having the Best Sex of my Life

- A Harvard Brain Researcher Warns You Against these Top 5 Deadly Brain-Destroying Habits

Even Barack Obama's op-ed about the war between Israel and Gaza seemed to get lost in the mix between "How to Write a Love Poem" and "How to Grieve an Estranged Parent." And how can anyone compete with sex? But seriously, I began to think about different ways medical narratives can (and should) appeal to readers. A good title helps, but I was able to come up with 20 additional properties – descriptive adjectives – that good narratives possess, in my opinion. Incorporating just a few of these elements in your essay, or coaching patients how to write theirs, will go a long way toward attracting readers:

1. **Engaging**: A medical narrative should captivate the reader's attention, encouraging them to continue reading.

2. **Informative**: It should provide valuable information about the patient's experience, disease progression, and treatment process.

3. **Empathetic**: The narrative should show understanding and compassion for the patient's situation, offering a humanistic perspective of medicine.

4. **Clear**: The language should be simple and straightforward, avoiding unnecessary medical jargon that could confuse the reader.

5. **Comprehensive**: It should cover relevant aspects of the patient's medical history – symptoms, diagnosis, treatment, and follow-up – and be clinically sound.

6. **Authentic**: The narrative should be truthful and honest, reflecting the realities of medical practice and patient care, including its shortcomings.

7. **Detailed**: It should include specific details that help the reader understand the patient's condition and the medical process but use plain language understandable to the average reader (see essay 14).

8. **Reflective**: It should encourage the reader to think deeply about the patient's experience and the role of medicine in addressing human suffering.

9. **Respectful**: The narrative should respect the patient's privacy and dignity and avoid any form of stigmatizing or discriminatory language.

10. **Inspiring**: It should inspire the reader to appreciate the value of medicine in improving human health and well-being.

11. **Insightful**: It should provide insights into the patient's feelings, thoughts, and experiences, helping the reader understand the human side of medicine.

12. **Well-structured**: It should have a logical structure that facilitates the reader's understanding, with a clear beginning, middle, and end.

13. **Personalized**: It should reflect the unique experiences and perspectives of the patient, avoiding a one-size-fits-all approach.

14. **Personified**: Narratives often give human characteristics to non-human entities. For example, a patient might say, "My cancer is an enemy I'm fighting," which can convey their determination and struggle.

15. **Balanced**: It should present a balanced view of the patient's situation, acknowledging both the positive and negative aspects of their medical journey.

16. **Evocative**: It should evoke emotions and stimulate the reader's mind, helping them to relate to the patient's situation.

17. **Ironical**: Narratives can highlight paradoxes or contradictions in a patient's experience or treatment.

18. **Metaphorical**: Comparisons between two unlike things that share common characteristic can help convey a patient's feelings or symptoms in a way that's more relatable or understandable.

19. **Symbolic**: Symbols can be used to represent ideas or qualities. For example, a patient might describe their pain as a "burning fire," symbolizing intense discomfort.

20. **Imaginative**: Narratives that create sensory impressions can help physicians understand a patient's experience in a more visceral way.

One of the essayists I most admired was the late television broadcaster Andy Rooney. His end-of-show segments on *60 Minutes* were thoughtful and often hilarious. He used satire and whimsy to engage his audience, as well as many of the above techniques, often ending his monologue with a punchline. Sometimes, I put myself in Rooney's shoes – for example, by saving the best line for last. In an essay titled "My Lucky Life" – Rooney's last appearance on *60 Minutes* – he complained to viewers about his unwelcomed fame. Rooney ended with a plea: "If you do see me in a restaurant, please, just let me eat my dinner." I, on the other hand, would be happy to give you my autograph anytime.

6.
Physician Writers and Writers Who are Physicians

Let's close the gap!

"Oh, I didn't know you're a writer," my neighbor said as I handed her a complimentary copy of my recently-published book.

"Not really," I replied. "I'm just a physician who likes to write."

The conversation ended, but later I began to think: What's the difference between a physician writer and a writer who is a physician? What should I say to somebody else who makes a comment like my neighbor? I should have a 30 second elevator speech prepared.

A physician writer and a writer who is a physician are not the same. They have different focuses and roles. Here is my elevator pitch.

A physician writer is a professional who primarily specializes in medicine, but also has the skills to write about medical topics. Their primary role is as a physician, diagnosing and treating patients, but they also write as an avocation or as part of their professional responsibilities. This could include writing research papers, case studies, articles for medical journals, or informational materials for patients. For example, Dr. Atul Gawande, a renowned surgeon, writes extensively on public health issues and has published several books on medical topics, including *Being Mortal* and *The Checklist Manifesto*.

On the other hand, a writer who is a physician is someone whose primary role or profession is writing, but who also happens to be a trained physician. This person might write novels, screenplays, essays, or articles that may or may not be about medical topics. Their medical background could provide a unique perspective or depth to their writing, but their main focus is on the craft of writing itself. An example is the late Dr. Michael Crichton, who was trained as a physician but is best known for his writing, including the science fiction novels *The Andromeda Strain* and *Jurassic Park*.

As my elevator descends, time permitting, I would expand on the list of physicians who are writers and writers who are physicians, as well as their works. My list would consist of at least ten authors in addition to Gawande and Crichton:

1. **Sir Arthur Conan Doyle**: Best known for his detective series featuring Sherlock Holmes, Doyle was a physician before he became a successful author.

2. **Anton Chekhov**: A physician by training, Chekhov is one of the greatest writers of short stories in history. Some of his famous works include *The Cherry Orchard* and *Three Sisters*.

3. **Robin Cook**: Trained in ophthalmology, Cook is known for his medical thrillers, including *Coma* and *Outbreak*.

4. **Khaled Hosseini**: Formerly a practicing internist, Hosseini wrote best-selling novels like *The Kite Runner* and *A Thousand Splendid Suns*.

5. **Abraham Verghese**: A Professor of Medicine at Stanford University, Verghese has written several best-selling books including *Cutting for Stone* and *My Own Country*.

6. **Tess Gerritsen**: A retired physician, Gerritsen is a best-selling author known for her medical and crime thrillers, including the Rizzoli & Isles series.

7. **Oliver Sacks**: A neurologist, Sacks wrote several books about his patients and their unique neurological disorders, including *The Man Who Mistook His Wife for a Hat* and *Awakenings*, which was made into a feature film.

8. **Siddhartha Mukherjee**: An oncologist, Mukherjee wrote *The Emperor of All Maladies: A Biography of Cancer*, which won the Pulitzer Prize.

9. **Paul Kalanithi**: A neurosurgeon who wrote *When Breath Becomes Air*, a memoir about his life and battle with lung cancer. The book was published posthumously and became a best-seller.

10. **Lewis Mehl-Madrona**: Trained in family medicine, psychiatry, and clinical psychology, Mehl-Madrona is author of the *Coyote* trilogy and has worked with Indigenous communities to explore how to bring their culture and healing traditions into health care.

I quickly jotted down these authors without trying to differentiate which category they belonged to, i.e., whether they were primarily physician writers or writers who are (or were) physicians. When I tried to separate them into one or either of the two categories, I had some difficulty because the distinction was nearly impossible to make – the lines between "physician writer" and "writer physician" became blurred.

Naturally, the first few authors that jumped out at me were mainly writers who happened to be trained as physicians. But what about, for example, Verghese and Gawandi and a few of the others who have had dual careers practicing as physicians and making a living by writing?

I faced a similar dilemma when I tried to categorize physicians who are musicians. I wrote a piece about physicians and their hobbies, and in the case of jazz pianist Denny Zeitlin, his music is inseparable from his role as a psychiatrist: he is both a psychotherapist and recording jazz artist, as he describes on his websites – one for his role as a psychiatrist and one for his career as a musician.

The tipping point that decides which category they belong to, I suppose, is the amount of time spent practicing versus writing (or playing music). When the time is roughly equal, I don't bother to make the distinction between roles. It's similar for physician executives. When they divide their time equally between seeing patients and managing administrative activities, the "physician" and the "executive" are one and the same. But when physicians assume high-level nonclinical careers, people tend to see them primarily as executives.

You may be asking: why does any of this matter? I would answer: because I believe all physicians are writers, just as my colleague Peter Angood, MD, believes all physicians are leaders. No doubt some physicians are more capable writers (and leaders) than others; closing the gap between practicing and writing is not only desirable, it is therapeutic for physicians and beneficial for their patients.

If you want to close the gap between practicing and writing, try these 10 tips:

1. **Develop a Writing Routine**: Physicians can set aside a specific time each day or week for writing, even if it's just for a few minutes. This can help them develop a writing habit. (Early morning works best for me.)

2. **Use Personal Experiences**: Physicians have a wealth of experiences to draw from in their practice. They can use these experiences to inform their writing, whether it's a medical article, a research paper, or a novel.

3. **Attend Writing Workshops and Seminars**: These can provide physicians with the tools and techniques they need to improve their writing skills.

4. **Collaborate with Other Writers**: Physicians can learn a lot from other writers, especially those who are also in the medical field. They can collaborate on projects, share ideas, and provide feedback on each other's work.

5. **Write for Medical Journals**: Physicians can start by submitting articles to medical journals. This can help them gain experience in writing and also establish their credibility as writers.

6. **Hire a Writing Coach or Editor**: A professional can provide feedback on their writing and help them improve.

7. **Take Advantage of Technology**: There are many software and apps available that can help with writing, such as grammar checkers, dictation software, and project management tools.

8. **Practice Reflective Writing**: Reflecting on their experiences and writing about them can help physicians become better writers. It can also help them process their experiences and gain a deeper understanding of their practice.

9. **Read Widely**: As discussed in essay 4, reading a variety of materials, not just medical literature, can help physicians improve their writing skills and expose them to different writing styles.

10. **Start a Blog or Write a Book**: Physicians can share their insights and experiences with a wider audience through a blog or a book. This can also help them establish a writing portfolio.

I was contacted by a physician who had been viewing my posts on the internet. He wrote, "[I] realize that some of our interests align. I am very interested in the power of storytelling and how it affects doctors, patients, and our healthcare system in general…I consider myself a writer who became a doctor."

When we finally spoke, I gave him my 30 second elevator speech, which was well-rehearsed by then.

7.
Using the Narrative to
Reconnect with Practice

"In our rush to find clinical solutions, we often overlook the power of narrative. It is through sharing and understanding stories that we can reconnect to our patients and ourselves."
– Paul Kalanithi

A physician wrote on LinkedIn that he is retiring after 27 years of practice. This primary care physician remarked, "Though not an easy decision, it was the right one for me. The thought of not continuing to serve my patients made it a very difficult decision. I will cherish the family-like relationships I built with them over the years. I look forward to the next chapter with the excitement of not knowing where it will lead me. Looking forward to new ventures and partnerships."

This physician listed 20 separate "experiences" in his LinkedIn profile, ranging from practicing OB/GYN to internal medicine, teaching at two medical schools, and working for two health insurance companies. He has worked with and published research about homeless people. He is an entrepreneur and a philanthropist and has founded several companies. He claims to be "rediscovering the essence of everything." He is in his early 50s.

I wrote to him and said, "Good luck in your encore career." An "encore career" refers to a second, meaningful career that an individual pursues later in life, often after retiring from their first career. For physicians, this could mean transitioning from active clinical practice to a new role that typically involves less stress and more flexibility, but still leverages their extensive medical knowledge and experience.

Examples of encore careers can be found in essay 21, such as medical consulting, writing and editing, nonprofit work, research, and health policy. Some physicians have forsaken medicine completely for wine making, coffee roasting, teaching, running a family business, and other pursuits totally distanced from medical practice or unrelated to the field of medicine.

There are many reasons behind the exodus of physicians from medicine. Briefly summarized, they include:

1. **Burnout**: The high-stress environment of healthcare can lead to burnout, resulting in physicians reducing their hours or leaving practice.

2. **Administrative Burden**: Physicians often spend a significant amount of time on paperwork, electronic charting, and administrative tasks, which can be overwhelming and take time away from patient care.

3. **Financial Pressure**: Lower reimbursements from insurance companies, combined with the high cost of maintaining a practice and repaying medical school debt, can make practicing medicine less financially viable.

4. **Work-Life Balance**: The high demands of a medical practice can make it difficult for physicians to maintain a healthy balance between their work obligations and home life.

5. **Regulatory Changes**: Changes in healthcare regulations can add additional stress and workload to physicians, making practice more challenging.

The implications of a depleted physician workforce are significant for both patients and society. With fewer physicians, patients may have difficulty accessing care. This could lead to longer wait times for appointments and potentially delay necessary treatment. If physicians are overworked due to a shortage of colleagues, the quality of care they provide may decrease. A physician shortage may result in higher healthcare costs. With fewer providers, the demand for their services could drive up prices. Fewer physicians could mean less capacity to respond to public health crises, like pandemics or natural disasters. Finally, areas with fewer resources, such as rural or low-income communities, could be hit hardest by a physician shortage, exacerbating existing health disparities.

As much as I support physicians who seek career alternatives to medical practice, I am the first to remind them that the grass in not always greener on the other side; it's just different. Before they take a leap of faith into unchartered waters, I am keen to remind physicians to make sure they are absolutely certain they have exhausted all remedies that would allow them to continue to practice. That being the case, I wish them well and offer resources to explore their encore career.

However, I have recently been adding one more item to physicians' checklists before they leave practice. I ask whether they have attempted writing narratives to counteract burnout or whatever is driving them away from medicine. This might seem like a silly idea, but there is mounting evidence that "by bridging the divides that separate physicians from patients, themselves, colleagues, and society, narrative medicine offers fresh opportunities for respectful, empathic, and nourishing medical care," according to Rita Charon, MD, PhD, a leader in the field.

Carolyn Roy-Bornstein, MD, is a retired pediatrician and the writer-in-residence at the Lawrence (Massachusetts) Family Medicine Residency program. She wrote: "Narrative medicine programs have been shown to build empathy, foster meaningful engagement, shape perspectives, and offer a shared space where deep moral values are shaped and cultivated. All of this will sustain the physician when facing the moral ambiguities inherent in our work. Narrative medicine provides a regular forum where clinicians can share mutual struggles and find common solutions." Roy-Bernstein has observed that the narrative approach enhances resilience, wisdom, creativity, and joy, including the possibility "of finding meaning in our work and locating the joy in our jobs again."

Here are few quotes by other famous physician authors who have reflected on the power of the narrative to help reconnect to practice:

- "The practice of medicine becomes more fulfilling when we allow ourselves to be touched by the stories of our patients. It is through these narratives that we truly connect with the art of healing." - Dr. Atul Gawande, Surgeon and Author.

- "Narrative Medicine is the practice of incorporating the patient's story into their treatment. It reconnects us to the patient as a person, not just a set of symptoms." - Dr. Abraham Verghese, Professor for the Theory and Practice of Medicine, Stanford University Medical School.

- "Using narratives in medicine allows us to see the person behind the patient. It brings empathy back into the consultation room and helps us to reconnect to the fundamental principles of medical practice." - Dr. Danielle Ofri, Associate Professor of Medicine, New York University.

- "In our technical world, we often forget that medicine is a human practice. Using narratives helps us to remember this and to reconnect with our patients on a deeper level." - Dr. Jerome Groopman, Dina and Raphael Recanati Chair of Medicine at Harvard Medical School.

Of course, overcoming burnout and other pressures that motivate physicians to seek alternative careers is not as simple as writing about patients and learning from the intellectual exploration of prose and poetry. The complete solution requires a host of structural changes and a formidable campaign by the medical establishment to provide resources to healthcare leaders to ease burnout, encourage help-seeking, and improve well-being among the entire workforce of healthcare providers. (See, for example, essay 28 and the CDC initiative to support hospitals as they address physician burnout.)

Narrative medicine has proven a viable tool to help medical students and residents through training, but whether it can sustain them through years of practice is questionable and requires formal research. Meanwhile, there is certainly no shortage of works of fiction and non-fiction that could inform, edify, and lend fulfillment and sustainability to individuals interested in pursuing medicine and remaining in the profession. Time and again we have witnessed narration's potential to empower doctors by turning their conflicting emotions into compassionate reflections on their patients' and colleagues' relationships. There is no reason to believe writing initiatives will not bear fruit that can be harvested for years to come.

8.
Physicians Face Legal and Ethical Challenges in Writing Narratives

It's important to maintain professional standards and ethical integrity when writing narratives.

A physician told me she loved writing about her encounters with patients before the HIPAA era, but once the privacy laws were enacted she basically gave up on writing narratives and instead began writing poetry. "Poems bypass HIPAA," she confided, because our patients' identities are not usually revealed in poems, whereas narratives may compromise confidentiality. Also, she reminded me that our recall of patients from years or decades ago may obscure vital events or cloud the accuracy of our stories, perhaps even obfuscating the truth, which is anathema to narrative medicine.

It is true that physicians who write medical narratives may encounter various legal and ethical challenges as they navigate the intersection of healthcare and creative expression. Because narrative medicine involves the use of storytelling and personal narratives to understand and enhance the patient experience, it raises considerations not only related to privacy and confidentiality, but also consent and professional boundaries. Many of these issues overlap. Here are a dozen challenges that physician authors of narrative medicine must consider in order to preserve the integrity of their writing and reputation:

1. **Patient Confidentiality and Privacy**: The primary legal and ethical challenge for physician authors is respecting patient confidentiality and privacy. This is protected under the Health Insurance Portability and Accountability Act (HIPAA) in the U.S. and similar laws in other countries. Physicians must ensure that they do not disclose any identifiable patient information without explicit consent.

2. **Accuracy and Integrity**: Anonymizing patient stories and altering details to prevent identification are common strategies to address privacy concerns. In doing so, however, authors must not stray so far from the truth and essence of the story so that it appears more like a work of fiction than creative nonfiction. Physician authors have an ethical responsibility to present truthful and authentic stories while avoiding exaggeration or distortion that could mislead readers. I could tell from my colleague's comments that she struggled with the possibility that her "selective memory" might alter the authenticity of the narrative, and switching to poetry would obviate this concern.

3. **Informed Consent**: If identifiable information is to be used, physicians must obtain informed consent from patients. This consent should be specific, indicating that the information will be used for a narrative medicine piece, and the potential consequences of this should be clearly communicated. The consent of family members should also be obtained if they are the subjects of narratives. Patients should have the option to decline participation without any impact on their medical care.

4. **Potential Harm**: Physicians must consider the potential harm that could come from sharing patient stories, even with consent. This could include emotional distress or stigmatization. They must ensure that their narratives are respectful and sensitive to the experiences and feelings of their patients. They should forewarn patients that once a narrative appears in

writing – anywhere – very rarely can it be retracted. This is important for patients to know, because sharing an experience with a doctor as opposed to seeing it in writing might evoke different reactions.

5. **Commercialization and Exploitation**: There is an ethical challenge surrounding the use of patient stories for profit. If a physician author publishes a book or sells their narrative medicine pieces, it may be seen as exploiting patient experiences for personal gain. Should the proceeds go to the author or be shared with the patient? Perhaps profits should be donated to an organization designated by the patient.

6. **Objectivity and Professionalism**: Physicians must maintain a balance between their professional responsibilities and their role as writers. They must ensure that their writing does not interfere with their clinical judgment or professional relationships. Dr. Denny Zeitlin, the psychiatrist and jazz musician whom I briefly mentioned in essay 6, wrote: "My musical activities have always remained subordinate to my primary responsibility to patients in my full-time practice and to trainees."

6. **Respect for Autonomy**: The patient's story is their own, and physicians should respect their autonomy in how it is told. They should avoid misrepresentation or manipulation of the patient's narrative to fit a particular theme or message. Honor the patient, always, as Dr. Rita Charon reminds us.

7. **Professional Boundaries:** Physician authors need to maintain appropriate professional boundaries when sharing personal narratives or engaging in narrative medicine. Avoiding the disclosure of sensitive personal details that could compromise the doctor-patient relationship is important. This is one of the reasons physicians have been cautioned about their use of social media: actions and content posted online may negatively affect their reputations among patients and colleagues, may have consequences for their medical careers (particularly for physicians-in-training and medical students), and can undermine public trust in the medical profession.

8. **Conflict of Interest:** Physicians who write about their experiences in healthcare must be mindful of potential conflicts of interest. Disclosures about financial interests or relationships that could influence the narrative should be transparent.

9. **Cultural Sensitivity:** Physicians need to be culturally sensitive when sharing patient narratives, respecting diverse backgrounds, beliefs, and values. Avoiding stereotypes and ensuring narratives are inclusive are also ethical considerations.

10. **Publication and Copyright Issues:** Physicians writing for publication may encounter copyright issues, particularly if the narrative includes contributions from patients or if it is part of collaborative work. Understanding and respecting copyright laws is important.

11. **Educational Use and Research:** If narratives are used for educational purposes or research, additional ethical considerations arise. Institutional review board (IRB) approval may be required, and adherence to research ethics guidelines and "good clinical practice" is essential.

12. **Patient Empowerment:** Ensuring that narratives contribute to patient empowerment rather than vulnerability is another ethical consideration. Patients should be portrayed respectfully and with dignity.

Navigating these legal and ethical challenges requires a thoughtful and conscientious approach from physician authors practicing narrative medicine. Clear communication, transparency, and a commitment to patient welfare are essential elements in maintaining the trust and ethical integrity of the narrative medicine practice. Physicians must always prioritize patient privacy and respect, balancing their dual roles as healthcare providers and storytellers.

9.
Reflections on the "Cut Throat" Nature of Medicine and (Maybe) Writing

Do you have what it takes to rise above the crowd?

I opined in essay 20 that future medical students will be of high caliber, and in the next essay I alluded to a survey that showed students were under tremendous pressure to excel. This led me to think about the different pathways taken by medical students and writers to achieve success, as well as how "success" is defined by physicians and writers. No doubt, doctors and writers have different concepts of "success."

Medical education is often described as "cut throat" due to the intense competition and high stakes involved, beginning in college and even beforehand. (Would you believe experts advise that future doctors should start prepping as early as age 7!) From the moment students enter pre-medical programs, they are faced with the pressure to outperform their peers to secure a spot in medical school. This competition continues throughout their education as they strive to excel in their studies, clinical rotations, and board exams.

The level of competition is primarily due to the limited number of slots available in medical schools and residency programs. These institutions also prioritize high grades, strong test scores, and impressive extracurricular activities, adding to the pressure on students to outshine in all areas. Moreover, the rigor and breadth of the curriculum, the long hours of study, and the emotional toll of clinical practice can make medical education a stressful and demanding journey.

On the other hand, the path to becoming a writer is a different kind of challenge. It is less structured and does not follow a fixed timeline or curriculum like medical education. Aspiring writers often face the challenge of developing their unique voice and style, honing their craft, and finding their niche in the market. Unlike medical education, there is no standardized measure of success or achievement in writing.

For example, at Sarah Lawrence College, which is in close proximity to the New York City literary scene, students in the MFA writing program "are evaluated through a combination of factors," according to Madeleine Mori, assistant program director (written correspondence, November 21, 2023). Mori stated: "Students do receive grades for each course, which has its own syllabus and grading rubric, largely comprised of written assignments and class participation/attendance, with sometimes presentations, and/or a final project or portfolio required for the course. Students enrolled in workshops are also given written evaluations by their instructors, a system of which students are quite fond here. They are generally quite encouraging/constructive and in-depth." (Disclosure: my son graduated the MFA writing program at Sarah Lawrence.)

Similarly, many medical schools have deemphasized traditional A-F grades and moved to a system of honors/pass/fail, or they offer the option of either grades or honors/pass/fail. If there's any doubt whether the cut throat culture of college persists in medical students once they enter medical school, consider the fact that many students opt for "letter" grades and eschew pass/fail grades even though pass/fail reduces student stress and anxiety and far outweighs any potential downsides. Some medical students, it seems, are incapable of becoming uncompetitive (see essay 38).

Also, consider the fact that writing students are encouraged to take classes outside their declared concentrations. At first glance, this seems to mirror how medical students are exposed to different clinical fields in their third and fourth years of medical school. But medical training is more parochial compared with the ethos that guides graduate writing programs. In reality, medical students are not exposed to even half of all the specialties and subspecialties in medicine, even factoring in their time in elective rotations in their final year of medical school.

If there is a cut throat culture among writers, it seems to me that it is more about attempting to stand out in a crowded market rather than outperforming peers on standardized exams. Writers often face rejection and criticism, which can be emotionally challenging. However, they also have more flexibility and autonomy in their work, allowing them to explore various genres and styles: fiction, poetry, creative nonfiction, and speculative fiction.

The path to becoming both a physician and a writer requires dedication, hard work, and resilience. However, the pressure and competition in medical education are more intense, resulting in a high degree of burnout and mental health disorders due to the pressures. The maladies seen in writers are often self-inflicted; writers tend to torment themselves with others' success, flagellate themselves with self-criticism, torture themselves with revisions, and constantly measure their worth by their publications.

Writers and physicians clearly want to be noticed, because the job market is limited. But doctors have no problems finding jobs as long as they aren't too picky about the offerings (the "match" seems to have eliminated much of the supply and demand problem). It is much more difficult for writers to support themselves solely by writing. They often resort to teaching or acquiring a menial day job while waiting to "hit it big." Writers face more financial instability and uncertainty than doctors; there's really no such thing as a "starving" doctor.

The path to becoming a successful writer can be circuitous – in medicine it's more straightforward – and success is often an individualistic pursuit, experienced personally by the writer, untethered from exams or a fixed set of criteria. Success as a writer can be defined in various ways, including publication, critical acclaim, or personal satisfaction. Success in writing can also come from finding a niche, building an audience, or creating unique and compelling content. Because medicine is team-based, success is measured by the contributions and efficiency of people working together for a common cause (i.e., the patient), and success is shared within the team and the organization.

Despite their differences, doctors and writers do have in common certain key aspects of training, such as persistence, commitment to their craft, and continuous learning. Ultimately, physicians and writers want to be recognized for their uniqueness and brilliance. If there is a red thread it might be their drive to rise above the competition.

10.
How Can Storytelling be Integrated with Medical Practice?

"Every person is a story that is trying to be told."
– Carl Jung

Storytelling is an ancient pastime. Stories can be found everywhere – from scripture to theatre – and sometimes combined into one medium, like the movie The Ten Commandments. Essentially, a story expresses how and why life changes. That's why stories are prime for the field of medicine: illness and sickness transform lives.

In addition, storytelling is interactive, as is medical practice. The interaction between a storyteller and one or more listeners is no different than that of a doctor who engages with patients, families, and trainees. The storyteller uses language and gestures meant to encourage the active imagination of the listeners involved in the presentation of a story – a narrative. There are many cultures and art forms, each with rich traditions, customs and opportunities for storytelling. Medicine is but one of them.

Storytelling can be a powerful tool in the field of medicine, enhancing practice in various ways – for example, by improving communication, fostering empathy, improving education, promoting adherence to treatment, providing therapeutic benefits, aiding in community outreach, and supporting research and advocacy efforts. Yet, from my perspective, physicians tell far too few stories, perhaps reserving them for gallows humor over lunch.

For sure, the hurried pace of practice and the assembly line treatment of patients (essay 23) are not conducive to storytelling. Also, storytelling is not top-of-mind with some physicians due to their extensive scientific training and inadequate exposure to the humanities (essay 4). However, physicians' interest in people in general creates a tremendous backdrop for storytelling. Here are a dozen ways in which storytelling can be integrated into medical practice:

1. **Doctor-Patient Relationship**: Storytelling can be used to improve the communication between patients and doctors. Patients often feel more comfortable sharing their symptoms, medical history, and concerns in the form of a narrative. This can provide doctors with more comprehensive information, aiding in diagnosis and treatment.

2. **Patient-Centered Care:** Encouraging patients to share their medical histories and experiences through storytelling can help healthcare professionals better understand the context of their illness. Sharing personal stories can help build trust between healthcare providers and patients, creating a more open and collaborative relationship.

3. **Medical Education:** Presenting medical information through case studies and narratives can make complex concepts more relatable and memorable for students. Using patient stories during clinical rounds can help medical students and residents develop a deeper understanding of the human side of medicine. Physicians need to be cognizant of "teachable moments," and substitute a good, lasting story for factual information that may soon be forgotten.

4. **Empathic Communication Skills:** Storytelling can help healthcare providers better understand the unique experiences and challenges of their

patients, helping them better connect with patients on an emotional level. Storytelling techniques can be employed to communicate difficult news in a compassionate and understandable manner.

5. **Health Promotion and Adherence:** Storytelling can be used to convey health messages effectively, making them more engaging and relatable to the target audience. Narratives can be powerful tools for motivating patients to adopt healthier lifestyles and adhere to treatment recommendations. Patients are more likely to follow a treatment plan they understand.

6. **Interprofessional Collaboration:** Sharing stories within healthcare teams can promote a sense of camaraderie and understanding among different professionals, fostering a collaborative and supportive work environment.

7. **Cultural Competence:** Storytelling can help bring to light the specific health issues and barriers faced by different cultural and socioeconomic groups, guiding the development of culturally sensitive interventions and policies. Stories can help healthcare professionals understand the cultural backgrounds and perspectives of their patients, leading to more culturally competent care.

8. **Quality Improvement:** Storytelling can be employed in root cause analysis to understand the context and contributing factors behind medical errors or adverse events, leading to more effective quality improvement initiatives.

9. **Research Dissemination:** Physicians can use storytelling to effectively present case studies and research findings. This can make their work more accessible and relatable to the general public, policymakers, and other healthcare professionals.

10. **Reducing Stigma:** Sharing stories can help raise awareness about stigmatizing conditions and encourage people to seek help and receive ap-

propriate treatment. Sharing stories of individuals living with stigmatized conditions can help reduce societal stigma and discrimination.

11. **Reducing Health Disparities:** Storytelling can simplify complex medical information and make it more understandable for everyone, regardless of their educational background or health literacy levels. This can help reduce disparities by ensuring everyone can access and understand crucial health information.

12. **Advocacy:** Physicians can use stories to advocate for their patients, particularly when it comes to securing funding for treatments or raising awareness about a particular condition.

Incorporating storytelling into medical practice requires a thoughtful and planned approach, respecting patient privacy and confidentiality. Training programs and workshops can help healthcare professionals develop effective storytelling skills and utilize them appropriately in various healthcare settings to achieve beneficial treatment outcomes.

11.
Overcoming Writer's Block

"Writing about a writer's block is better than not writing at all."
– Charles Bukowski

Bob Dylan took a seat at the piano at a concert in Philadelphia during the seventh leg (Fall 2023) of his two-year worldwide "Rough and Rowdy Ways" tour. He claimed to be at a loss for words. "What's the matter with me?" he asked. "I don't have much to say."

Those are the opening lines of "Watching the River Flow," the 1971 song that appeared on his "Greatest Hits Vol. II" album. The song is allegedly about finding peace with writer's block. I have difficulty believing that Dylan was blocked. More likely, as legend has it, the lyrics were hastily written in a New York recording studio with backing musicians in tow impatiently waiting to lay down a tune.

Drummer Jim Keltner recalled, "I remember Bob ... had a pencil and a notepad, and he was writing a lot. He was writing these songs on the spot in the studio, or finishing them up at least." Writer's block? Ha, ha! What some authors would give to be as prolific as Dylan.

"Watching the River Flow" captured Dylan at a time of transition from delivering less politically engaged material to finding a new balance between his public and private life, wishing to avoid culture clashes and instead sit back to watch the disagreements play themselves out: like watching the river flow.

Writer's block has likely existed since the dawn of writing, but the term itself was only coined in 1947 by the famous psychiatrist Edmund Bergler. In 1950, Bergler published a paper titled "Does 'Writer's Block' Exist?" He answered in the affirmative and labeled writer's block a "neurotic disease."Norman Mailer quipped, "Writer's block is only a failure of the ego," suggesting that all writing problems are psychological problems, stemming primarily from a fear of being judged.

The truth is, writer's block can be brought on by various factors, including stress, self-doubt, lack of inspiration, or external pressures. Paraphrasing J.K Rowling, the thing that is most wonderful and terrifying to writers is a blank page. She and many authors are all too familiar with the situation where an individual, particularly a writer, is unable to produce new work or experiences a creative slowdown. Every writer's been there; it's inevitable, really. Many have shared their experiences and strategies for overcoming it. Here are a few suggestions from physicians who have become stuck at writing:

Danielle Ofri, MD, PhD, shared that her writing process includes periods of frustration and stagnation. She emphasized that writing is hard work and often requires pushing through these difficult periods.

Atul Gawande, MD, MPH, has talked about the importance of discipline and routine in writing. He sets aside specific times for writing and sticks to this schedule, which can help push through periods of low inspiration or productivity.

Suzanne Koven, MD, MFA, a primary care physician and writer-in-residence at Massachusetts General Hospital, has discussed how she uses her experiences with patients to fuel her writing. When facing writer's block, drawing from real-life experiences can provide a wealth of material.

Abraham Verghese, MD, MFA, said in an interview that writing, much like medicine, requires practice and dedication. He suggested that persistent writing, even when it feels challenging, can help overcome periods of writer's block.

A good overview of writer's block was published by Patricia Huston, MD, MPH in *Canadian Family Physician*. Here are some insights gleaned from that article:

1. **Embrace the Process**: Many physician authors emphasize the importance of viewing writing as a process, not a one-time event. They suggest accepting writer's block as a normal part of that process – not a failure – and breaking down the work into small, manageable tasks.

2. **Write Regularly**: Physician authors often recommend establishing a regular writing routine, even in the midst of a busy medical practice. This helps to keep the writing muscles strong and can help overcome periods of block.

3. **Use Clinical Experiences as Inspiration**: As physicians, they often draw on their clinical experiences for inspiration. This can help to bypass writer's block as they always have a rich source of stories and ideas from their daily practice.

4. **Peer Support and Collaboration**: Some physician authors find that discussing their ideas with colleagues or co-authors can help break through periods of writer's block. This can provide fresh perspectives and stimulate new ideas.

5. **Continuing Education and Learning**: Physician authors are lifelong learners. Engaging in ongoing education, attending conferences, or read-

ing medical literature can provide new ideas and inspiration, helping to overcome writer's block. Education has been my salvation. I told my narrative medicine instructor that one of the reasons I wanted to enroll in the program was to be exposed to new material that I could incorporate into my writing. To my surprise, the class discussions proved more bountiful!

6. **Mindfulness and Stress Management**: Physician authors also recognize the impact of stress on creativity. Many recommend mindfulness practices, such as meditation or yoga, to manage stress and maintain mental clarity, thereby helping to overcome writer's block.

Here are 10 additional strategies that have helped writers deal with writer's block:

1. **Routine and Discipline**: Get your brain into the habit of producing creative work at specific times.

2. **Change of Environment**: A different setting can stimulate creativity. Try changing your workspace or writing outdoors.

3. **Free Writing**: Set a timer for a specific amount of time and write continuously without worrying about grammar, punctuation, or making sense. This can help you get the creative juices flowing.

4. **Physical Activity**: Exercise can stimulate brain activity and reduce stress, potentially helping to overcome writer's block.

5. **Mind Mapping**: This technique involves writing down a central idea and creating a web of related ideas around it. It can help to organize your thoughts and stimulate creativity.

6. **Avoid Perfectionism**: Don't pressure yourself to write perfectly in the first draft. Allow yourself to write poorly, knowing you can revise and improve later.

7. **Take Breaks**: Overworking can lead to burnout and block creativity. Make sure to take regular breaks, relax, and recharge.

8. **Derive Inspiration from Other Sources**: Reading a book, watching a movie, or listening to music can provide inspiration and help to overcome writer's block.

9. **Address Imposter Syndrome**: If you feel like you are not really a writer, play with the idea and write like you are someone else. Psychologists call this "paradoxical intervention" – achieving a desired result by engaging in opposite behavior.

10. **Break it Down**: Mark Twain famously said, "The secret of getting ahead is getting started. The secret of getting started is breaking your complex overwhelming tasks into small manageable tasks, and starting on the first one."

When I draw a blank at writing, I just "Let it Be." I occupy my time with something else, usually listening to music. I don't worry about not being able to write. Hugh MacLeod, author of *Ignore Everybody*, observed: "Writer's block is just a symptom of feeling like you have nothing to say, combined with the rather weird idea that you should feel the need to say something. Why? If you have something to say, then say it. If not, enjoy the silence while it lasts. The noise will return soon enough."

Of course, Dylan's comments to the Philadelphia concert-goers were not meant to be serious. At 82, at the tail end of a monumental career, he still has plenty to write about as well as a justified belief that his new material stands tall alongside the pillars of his celebrated catalog. *The Guardian* cited "Rough and Rowdy Ways" for its "deep musical and lyrical erudition, witticisms and considerable panache." *Pitchfork* called it a "gorgeous and meticulous record." And *Rolling Stone* said "it's an absolute classic."

I'd be happy with those reviews of my writing at any stage of my career, let alone in my ninth decade, should I live that long!

12.
Those Dreaded Creative Differences

Daryl Hall is trying to stop John Oates from selling a portion of the publishing rights to the duo's catalog of songs. No can do!

Say it isn't so! Daryl Hall is suing John Oates. The best-selling pop duo of all time, singing and songwriting partners since their college days at Temple University in the early 1970s, are embroiled in a bitter business dispute. In November 2023, Hall filed a lawsuit in a Nashville court arguing that Oates' plan to sell his share of a joint venture would violate a business agreement between them.

Hall was seeking an order preventing the sale of Oates' stake of Whole Oats Enterprises to Primary Wave Music, the music publishing company that owns rights to the catalogs of Prince, Stevie Nicks, and Alice Cooper, as well as rights to pioneering rock and blues label Sun Records. Primary Wave has already owned significant interest in Hall and Oates' song catalog for more than 15 years.

Business differences between Hall and Oates have also brought their creative differences to light. A year before the lawsuit was filed, Hall disparaged Oates on Bill Maher's "Club Random" podcast, saying, "You think John Oates is my partner? … He's my business partner. He's not my creative partner."

He continued, "John and I are brothers, but we are not creative brothers. We are business partners. We made records called Hall & Oates together, but we've always been very separate, and that's a really important thing for me."

Hall then went on to diminish the collaborative aspect of Hall & Oates, using the duo's 1980 smash hit "Kiss on My List" as an example of their apparent creative separation. "I did all those [harmonies]," Hall said. "That's all me." Oates is not credited as a songwriter on "Kiss on My List," but is listed as a co-producer with Hall.

Hall's split with Oats may not have the magnitude of the breakup of, say, Lennon and McCartney or Simon & Garfunkel, but it does demonstrate how those dreaded creative differences can crop up in in the writing business, particularly songwriting.

Although writing is often considered a solitary activity, with many writers preferring to work alone, this is not a hard and fast rule. Some writers thrive in collaborative environments and often choose to work with partners. Writing partnerships can provide a sounding board for ideas, a source of inspiration, and a way to share the workload.

Examples of successful writing teams include Terry Pratchett and Neil Gaiman, who co-wrote *Good Omens*, which was turned into a British fantasy comedy television series, and Nicci French, a pseudonym for the husband-and-wife team Nicci Gerrard and Sean French. Their acclaimed psychological thrillers have sold more than sixteen million copies around the world.

In the realm of screenwriting, partnerships are even more common. Many television shows and films are written by teams who brainstorm ideas, develop plots and characters, and write scripts together. However, writing partners who engage in creative writing can have differences based on their individual styles, perspectives, writing processes, and preferences. These differences can manifest in several ways:

1. **Writing Style**: Each writer has a unique writing style, which may clash with their partner's preferences. One partner may prefer a descriptive, elaborate style, while the other might favor a concise, straightforward approach.

2. **Story Development**: Writers may have different ideas about the direction the story should take, the tone, or the overall message. One writer may excel at crafting compelling characters, while the other may shine in plot development or setting descriptions.

3. **Writing Process**: Some writers are planners who outline everything before they start, while others are more spontaneous, letting the story evolve as they write (see the preceding essay).

4. **Genre Preference**: One partner may enjoy writing fantasy or science fiction, while the other may be more inclined towards mystery or romance.

5. **Work Habits**: Some writers prefer structured schedules and deadlines, while others may thrive in a more flexible environment. One writer may be a morning person, finding their most productive time is at the break of dawn, while the other may be a night owl, doing their best work in the late hours.

6. **Communication Preferences:** For example, one partner prefers detailed written feedback, while the other prefers face-to-face discussions.

7. **Handling Criticism:** Writers may have different sensitivities to criticism or different approaches to providing feedback. They have not created a safe space for open dialogue about improvements.

8. **Roles and Responsibilities:** Writers may have different expectations regarding who handles specific aspects of the writing process (e.g., drafting, editing, marketing).

9. **Flexibility:** One partner may be more open to changes and revisions, while the other may prefer sticking to the initial plan.

Successful writing partnerships require ongoing communication, mutual respect, and a willingness to compromise. If you are part of a writing team, consider the following options to resolving differences with your partner:

1. **Open Communication**: Discuss your individual strengths, weaknesses, and preferences openly. Understand each other's work habits and respect them. Establishing open and honest communication from the start and checking in regularly on the partnership and addressing any issues promptly signals you are willing to adapt to the problem.

2. **Compromise**: Embrace flexibility and compromise. Understand that creative projects often evolve, and being open to adjustments can lead to a stronger end product. Regularly discuss and agree on any significant changes to avoid misunderstandings. Find a middle ground where both of you can agree. This could be a blend of your styles, alternating between who leads on character development or plot, or setting a shared writing schedule that suits both of you.

3. **Division of Labor**: Clearly define roles and responsibilities early on. Acknowledge each other's strengths and interests and assign tasks accordingly. Regularly reassess and make adjustments as needed. Paradoxically, embracing your differences can enhance the creativity and richness of your joint work.

4. **Regular Feedback**: Establish a routine for providing constructive feedback. This will help both of you grow and improve your writing skills, ensuring the final product is a true collaborative effort.

5. **Mutual Respect**: Respect each other's creative process and ideas. Establish a constructive feedback process. Focus on the work rather than personal attributes. Learn to appreciate each other's differences. Remember, the goal is to create a cohesive piece of work that reflects both of your voices.

6. **Accommodation:** Establish clear expectations and timelines. Discuss and agree upon a workflow that accommodates each other's working styles. Regular check-ins can help hold each accountable to the other.

7. **Professional Editing**: Consider hiring a professional editor who can provide an objective perspective and help blend your distinct styles into a cohesive whole.

After a 50+ year partnership, you would have thought that Hall & Oates had learned to define the goals and themes of their projects from the beginning, and that they regularly revisited and discussed the overarching vision to ensure both songwriters were on the same page (no pun intended) – creatively and business-wise. At this juncture, I doubt they will ever be able to compromise and find common ground. Hall seems vehement in moving forward with his lawsuit, which has gone to arbitration. I can't go for that!

13.
Bad Grammar Makes Me Mad.
I Can't Help It.

Ensuring your prose is grammatically correct and free of errors involves a combination of self-editing techniques, leveraging technology, and seeking feedback.

Some of the most brilliantly funny men have the saddest personal lives. John Belushi, Chris Farley, and Sam Kinison were all preceded by Jerome Lester Horwitz, otherwise known as Curly of the Three Stooges: n'yuk-n'yuk-n'yuk. Why, soitenly the tragic life of a comedic legend deserves a great biography, and while Curly's niece (Moe's daughter) did her best to amass a wealth of Curly memorabilia – a mixture of written material and rare photographs of Curly's family, films, and personal life – the book was poorly written and edited, and it contained multiple spelling and grammar errors. According to the author, "I wrote this in less than 90 days," and it definitely shows.

If it makes your blood boil when you read prose punctuated incorrectly and containing bad grammar, you are not alone. A study from researchers at the University of Birmingham found that, when certain people come across grammar errors, their bodies respond physically. Departures from linguistic normality (i.e., errors in grammar, syntax, and punctuation) trigger a clear cardiovascular reaction – decreased heart rate variability, which may signal several potential health issues – and the cardiovascular response becomes stronger as the writing violations become more frequent.

The researchers also discovered that the physiological responses were less severe when the study subjects had to deal with grammatical mistakes spoken by someone with a foreign accent (in this case, Polish). Listening to a foreign speaker didn't itself affect the subjects' heart rate. That suggests participants, who were British, expected a non-native speaker to make more grammatical mistakes and were more forgiving of those mistakes.

The study was conducted so that 41 healthy, British English-speaking adults listened to 40 English speech samples, half of which contained grammatical errors. The texts were read in a native British and a Polish accent by both a male and a female voice. Participants were instructed to listen to the four different speakers in both error-free and error-ridden conditions. Listening to speech containing errors reduced heart rate variability, and the reduction tended to be proportional to the number of mistakes.

The authors concluded: "The observation brings into focus a new dimension of the intricate relationship between physiology and cognition, suggesting that cognitive effort reverberates through the physiological system in more ways than previously thought." In other words, becoming upset at someone who uses bad grammar is reflexive. It's in our DNA. It can feel like an assault on our system.

No wonder misplaced apostrophes make me angry. I live in Charlotte, home to Bojangles, a restaurant chain founded in 1977 and known for its "chicken 'n biscuits," now served at over 800 locations in 15 states. Fans from all over know Bojangles for their catchy tagline – "It's Bo Time!" However, the company has been too chicken to even say where the apostrophe in its name is supposed to go. Is it Bojangle's or Bojangles' – or simply Bojangles without an apostrophe? Over time, the final apostrophe has migrated several times.

Actually, at one time, the official Bojangles logo included an apostrophe flat above the S – not before or after. "The only plausible explanation," according to The Grammarian, otherwise known as Jeffrey Barg, "is that the restaurant chain couldn't decide whether the apostrophe was supposed to go before or after the S, so it split the difference like splitting a perfectly flaky biscuit."

The restaurant was initially spelled "Bojangle's," like McDonald's. In its most recent incarnation, there is no apostrophe. The punctuation free logo is clearly at odds with rules for the use of possessive apostrophes (don't get me started on the 'n). To make matters worse, the "j" in Bojangles is dotted by a five-point star rather than a *tittle*, which is the name of the small distinguishing mark (the dot) that should appear over a lowercase *i* (and a lowercase *j*).

At least there is no confusing the restaurant with the song, "Mr. Bojangles," written by Jerry Jeff Walker, a 1970 hit for the Nitty Gritty Dirt Band and a favorite of Sammy Davis Jr.'s. But hold the gravy 'n biscuits. The restaurant's founders *did* name the establishment after the song. It came to them as they were driving along the highway and heard it, according to Jackie Woodward, formerly the chief marketing officer at Bojangles. Furthermore, in an interview with *The Washington Post*, Woodward confessed: "What makes my job so much fun is that people do care about whether Bojangles has an apostrophe or not. It shows the passion that our customers have for our food."

I don't pretend to be a culinary expert or an expert in linguistics, but obvious grammar mistakes rile me. They are visible to everyone, and egregious errors indicate a lack of fundamental knowledge and/or proofreading. That's why I am so grateful for professional editors – they've saved my hide countless times. One that I have worked closely with jokingly told me that she spends her time "placing missing commas." Another editor told me she could reduce my word count by "taking out slivers [of words], like a fine surgeon's scalpel," and I wouldn't notice anything was missing!

Apart from proofreading your work and consulting an editor, there are many ways to ensure your prose is grammatically correct and free of errors and mistakes:

1. **Use Automated Tools**: There are many online tools and software programs available that can help in checking the grammar and spelling mistakes. Tools like Grammarly, Hemingway Editor, ProWritingAid, Ginger, etc. can be quite helpful. Microsoft Word's built-in spelling and grammar check can catch many common mistakes.

2. **Read Aloud**: The study referred to above implies that, by reading your work out loud, you can often catch errors that you might miss when reading silently. This method can help you identify awkward sentences or phrases, missing words, and other errors.

3. **Peer Review**: Share your work with a friend, colleague, or writing group. They might catch errors that you overlooked.

4. **Take a Break**: After writing, take a break – hours to days – before reviewing your work. This will help you see your work from a fresh perspective and you will be more likely to catch any errors.

5. **Print It Out**: Sometimes, reading a physical copy can make it easier to spot mistakes, as opposed to viewing it on a computer screen.

6. **Use a Style Guide**: Style guides, like the APA or AMA manual of style, provide rules for grammar, punctuation, and syntax. They can be a valuable resource for ensuring your writing is grammatically correct. Also, styles vary. It's been drilled into college students that they should know which style they're meant to be using when writing their papers, e.g., Chicago or MLA.

7. **Practice Regularly**: The more you write, the better you get. Regular practice can help you improve your grammar and reduce the number of errors in your writing.

8. **Read More**: Reading well-written books, articles, and papers and modeling their style can help you improve your grammar and writing skills.

9. **Attend Writing Workshops or Courses**: These can help you to improve your writing skills and learn more about grammar and punctuation.

10. **Use a Dictionary and Thesaurus**: These tools can help you choose the correct words, find alternatives and synonyms, and avoid repetition, which can improve the quality of your writing.

11. **Don't Make Assumptions**: Your mind can easily trick you into thinking something is there when it isn't. Proofread your work closely; don't rush through it.

Despite his mispronunciations, Curly had an uncanny ability to instantly spell big words, such as "chrysanthemum," if asked. The gag was that he never did it when something important was at stake. But your writing *is* important. Don't become a victim of soikemstance by not asking for editorial help. Indubitably!

INSPIRATION

14.
The Importance of Plain Language in Medical Practice

Find common ground in the doctor-patient relationship.

Comedy legend Joan Rivers was best known for asking her audiences "Can we talk?" – a euphemism for miscommunication and misunderstanding between people. Several experiences early in my career taught me the value of communicating with patients on their terms. I fear many doctors learn this lesson the hard way, because medical training emphasizes the importance of diagnosis and treatment, often neglecting interpersonal and cultural aspects of the doctor-patient relationship.

I found this to be true in my third year of medical school, soon after I began my clinical clerkships. I was working in the emergency department (ED) of a children's hospital, and I was evaluating a child with a rash. I was pretty sure the rash was impetigo, and after getting a thumb's up from the ED attending, I blurted to the father, "Your daughter has impetigo."

The father became concerned, and in a worried tone asked, "Can you break that down for me?" I didn't stop to think about the consequences of my actions – diagnosing his daughter in a straightforward manner by sight alone, without taking a history, and using a diagnostic term he did not comprehend. I should have listened to his concerns and then explained she had a common rash seen in children her age, that it was called impetigo, and it was easily treatable.

I talked way over his head and caused unnecessary alarm. I vowed never to let that happen again. Since the incident, I made conscious attempts to use plain language with patients and families. If appropriate, I also made "small talk" to try and put patients at ease.

It wasn't until my final year in medical school, however, that I fully appreciated the fact that communication is a two-way street. I was making progress in relating to patients on their level, but it didn't occur to me that patients may have a language all their own that *I* may not understand.

One day I was evaluating a man in his late 50s. He had diabetes, and his glucose was poorly controlled. I had a conversation with him about how to take better control of his blood sugar. I made a few modifications to his therapy (with the approval of my preceptor), and then I asked whether he had any questions.

"Well doc," he replied, "can you help me with my nature?"

I looked at the man incredulously and asked him to repeat the question.

"My nature – what can you do for my nature," the man repeated.

I simply didn't understand, and I asked him once more to explain. I could tell he was becoming frustrated and angry, so I left the exam room and summoned my preceptor. My preceptor told me that the term "nature" was commonly used by men in his culture as a synonym for sexual functioning. The patient was trying to tell me he had erectile dysfunction, most likely due to diabetes.

Rather than spare the gentleman embarrassment, I added to it through my lack of cultural awareness and insensitivity to his anguish. I learned that patients may attach special meaning to symptoms and suffering. If I was to become a good doctor, I had to better understand the contexts of meaning for interpreting illness.

My final lesson in communication occurred when I was a first-year resident working in a "walk-in" clinic – a section of the ED designated for non-emergent medical problems. I picked up the patient's chart and read the chief complaint: "sore on head." I opened the exam room door and introduced myself, simultaneously scanning the young man's head for a sore. I didn't see it.

"Show me the sore," I said to the patient. He nonchalantly dropped his pants and pulled down his underwear to show me the sore on his "head."

"Oh, that head!" The situation called for penicillin – not a bandage.

The Plain Writing Act of 2010 requires the federal government to issue public documents, such as tax returns, federal college aid applications, and Veterans Administration forms, in simple, easy-to-understand language. The Act defines "plain writing" as "writing that is clear, concise, well-organized and follows other best practices appropriate to the subject or field and intended audience." Because medical practice is highly regulated by the government, it can be argued that the requirement to use plain language extends to physicians, especially their written communications and instructions to patients.

Of course, there are times when it may not be possible or even desirable to use plain language – for example, when dictating medical reports, operative notes, and consultations to other physicians. However, this does not excuse errors in documents due to unintelligible dictation or technical terms "lost in translation" during transcription. Medical records should be reviewed and corrected when they contain inaccuracies or missing fields.

Imagine my surprise after reading a patient's history in which it was reported she had made a suicide "jester" (instead of gesture). Such mistakes are no laughing matter. Hundreds of thousands of people die each year due to medical errors resulting from miscommunication. Improving communication between doctors, and between doctors and patients, is at the root of virtually all quality improvement initiatives.

The internet has made it easy for professional organizations and physicians to communicate and share information quickly to reach millions of people. However, a *JAMA* study showed that patient education materials contained in the websites of 16 medical specialties were either too complex or suffered from a lack of readability, making them difficult for patients to comprehend and potentially contributing to poor health.

I'd like to think that, if I decide to practice again, my experiences as a younger physician, plus those in industry, will have strengthened my communication skills. I've learned valuable lessons at the bedside as well as writing educational material for patients while working in the pharmaceutical industry, including information destined for consumers searching the Internet.

I use simple words and phrases. I aim for a sixth grade reading level. I avoid the use of unfamiliar scientific or medical terms, and I never use complex language or, alternatively, language that "dumbs down" information to the point where medical accuracy is lost. It is important to strike the right balance between simplicity and complexity by providing patients sufficient yet not overly detailed information.

Patients want answers to their problems delivered in a clear, unhurried manner. Overly scientific and technical medical explanations tend to create fear, anxiety, or confusion, causing a disconnection in the doctor-patient relationship. It's not uncommon for patients to discard information they find unusable, ultimately creating more work for physicians to develop positive relationships.

The answer to Joan Rivers' exhortation "Can we talk?" is "Yes" if doctors appear concerned and interested, take the time to listen before pronouncing judgment, attempt to understand symptoms as patients experience them, and translate the language of medicine into terms patients can understand.

15.
So, You Want to Go to Medical School!

Even with a criminal past, it's possible.

Over the years, I have mentored medical students, residents, and early-career physicians on various issues ranging from wellness to career choices. One of the memorable students I mentored was a 26-year-old undergraduate student who had entered his senior year in college in 2021 and was applying to medical schools for the 2022 incoming class.

The student had a 4.0 GPA, 515 Medical College Admission Test (MCAT) score (90th percentile), and stellar references, including one from the president of his college. His interpersonal skills were excellent. He was definitely "worthy to serve the suffering."

The problem is, in 2015, the student had a serious addiction to opioids and was arrested on a felony residential burglary (no one was harmed). He believed he was fortunate to have been arrested because through the legal system, he was able to receive months of overdue rehabilitative treatment.

It was during treatment that the student first realized his passion for helping other individuals. He is in recovery and has an entirely new lease on life. His criminal record has been expunged. Even so, the student felt uneasy about answering "no" to medical school application questions that inquired about the commission of a felony. He recognized there could be repercussions by answering in the negative – for example, if his history was ever uncovered or his fingerprints inadvertently remained in the system even though his record was expunged.

To help the student decide whether to disclose his felony on the secondary applications, I sought the advice of three deans of U.S. medical schools. I asked them to draw on their experience with applicants in similar situations. None of the deans were affiliated with medical schools to which the student had applied. All three deans independently agreed that the student should disclose the nature of his felony. I also consulted one other individual – an authority on physicians' mental health issues – and he agreed with the deans.

I shared the feedback with the student. He decided to disclose his felony conviction, reasoning that failure to do so could have resulted in an offer of admission being rescinded if the omission were discovered, or he could have been disenrolled from medical school if the omission were discovered sometime later.

In the application, the student included a letter from his attorney explaining the nature of the crime, its legal disposition, and the attorney's opinion: "It would not be a falsification on an employment or educational application for [the student] to answer 'no' to a question asking whether he has been convicted of a felony, or otherwise not disclosing this case when asked about his conviction record."

The student was granted interviews at several medical schools, and he was accepted into the medical school of his first choice. He aspires to become a psychiatrist practicing in a rural area.

A *US News & World Report* article concluded, "Applying to medical school seems hard enough; with a criminal record it can be doubly so. The best way to deal with this issue is by explaining what happened and why, lessons you learned, and steps you've taken to ensure it will not be repeated."

This was clearly the consensus among the medical school deans, i.e., applicants should be truthful and honest and disclose a past history of criminal activity when asked. (Students are under no obligation, however, to voluntarily disclose past criminal behavior if they are not asked about it.)

Some students choose to make their crime the focus of their personal comments essay, as suggested by the deans, whereas others choose to address it on secondary applications, as did the student discussed here. He wrote, in part, "As a result of this extreme, unorthodox, and shameful past, I have developed my passion for helping others. I plan to use my empathy to serve as a physician dedicated to treating all patients with respect and dignity."

Students who are forthcoming about their prior criminal activities may actually enhance their application to medical school if they can demonstrate in their essays that they have undergone a personal transformation that reflects positively on their personality, professionalism, and current lifestyle choices.

The student is aware of the challenges a prior conviction will have on his pursuit of a medical career. After he completes medical school, it is possible that his felony conviction, although expunged, will be revisited by states' medical licensing boards by virtue of the open-ended nature of the questions asked on licensing applications, which may ignore or supplant any legal argument or disposition.

In addition, a felony conviction can restrict or prohibit employment opportunities. The substantial investment required to become a doctor can be erased by a prior criminal conviction, even if that conviction has been expunged. Thus, the value of hiring a seasoned, experienced and highly qualified attorney to assist individuals through the maze of considerations

– from applying to medical school through applying to a job – cannot be understated

To produce the healthcare professionals and medical researchers that society needs, diversity and inclusion efforts in medical schools and residency training programs must be championed. It is encouraging that medical schools are reporting increases in enrollment in first-year Black and ethnic minority students. However, medical schools have yet to accord individuals recovered from substance use and mental health disorders similar parity.

Although this student's acceptance into medical school suggests that past criminal behavior can be eclipsed by present character, the MCAT remains a normative marker in medical school admissions. Without an accomplished academic record, he likely would not have been considered a viable candidate for medical school and rejected on the basis of his qualifications alone.

16.
The Real Story Behind Woodstock is Not the Brown Acid

If you can remember the 60s, you weren't there!

In my search for ever obscure rock music from my generation – not the greatest generation but the flower generation – I came across a CD collection of rare songs titled "Brown Acid: The Seventeenth Trip," appropriately sub-titled: "Heavy Rock from the Underground Come-down." The record review began as follows: "Lucky number 17? You better believe it. We here at Brown Acid have been scouring the high-ways and byways of America for even more hidden stashes of psych/garage/proto-punk madness from the so-called Aquarian Age. There's no flower power here, though – just acid casualties, rock stompers and major freakouts."

I pride myself on knowledge of rock and roll music (see essay 24, for example), so how did I miss the release of the previous 16 "trips?" It was because the record label that produces these gems (RidingEasy Records) focuses on heavy psych, doom, and metal, and is home to Monolord, Electric Citizen, Salem's Pot, Mondo Drag, Brown Acid Comps, Slow Season, The Well, Shooting Guns, R.I.P., Dunbarrow, Danava and many more lesser known bands that are not my style.

Nevertheless, psychedelia seems to be everywhere these days, especially in my field of psychiatry, where hallucinogens are front and center in psychiatric R&D and there are now FDA-approval agents for depressive disorders (although they are quite expensive). Psychiatrists and other "helpers" (not necessarily healers) began dabbling with hallucinogenic drugs in the 1960s, lending their name in part to the "turn on, tune in, drop out" counterculture popularized by LSD guru Timothy Leary, a Harvard psychologist. Hallucinogens have been used for centuries for spiritual purposes, shamanism, and healing. We are now seeing a resurgence of interest in their therapeutic potential.

Several studies have shown that hallucinogens, particularly psilocybin and LSD, may be effective in treating mental health disorders such as depression, anxiety, post-traumatic stress disorder (PTSD), and addiction. They appear to work by disrupting patterns of thought and allowing patients to have transformative experiences. Some hallucinogens may promote neuroplasticity, or the brain's ability to form new connections and change its structure and function. This could potentially be harnessed for therapeutic benefits. For example, psilocybin, found in "magic mushrooms," has been used in clinical trials to treat existential anxiety related to terminal illness. Patients have reported significant reductions in anxiety and depression, often after just one or two sessions.

Other hallucinogens, like ketamine and its "sinister" enantiomer, S-ketamine, have shown promise in treating postpartum depression, treatment-resistant depression, and depression with suicidal ideation, sometimes providing relief from symptoms within hours of use. Ketamine exerts its activity on the brain primarily through its actions on the N-methyl-D-aspartate (NMDA) glutamate receptor (glutamate is the major excitatory neurotransmitter in the brain). NMDA receptor antagonism causes complex "downstream" effects and is believed to be the mechanism of action underlying the antidepressant effects of ketamine. However, multiple other NMDA receptor antagonists have failed to demonstrate antidepressant efficacy, suggesting additional neural pathways are involved.

While early results are promising, there are few long-term studies on the safety and effectiveness of hallucinogens. Many hallucinogens are classified as Schedule I drugs, meaning they are illegal and considered to have no medical value. This makes it difficult to conduct research and limits access to potential treatments. While hallucinogens are generally not considered addictive, they can be misused. They can also potentially lead to dangerous behavior, particularly if used without medical supervision.

Some people may have negative reactions to hallucinogens, including panic, paranoia, and psychosis. There is also the risk of triggering latent mental health problems. Due to their illegal status, there is no standardization or quality control for hallucinogens. This means that users can't be certain of the strength or purity of what they're taking.

So, while hallucinogenic drugs show promising therapeutic benefits, their limitations and potential risks should not be overlooked. More research is needed to fully understand their potential and to develop safe and effective treatment protocols.

That's the scientific overview. Here's the mythical one.

Those of us belonging to the "Woodstock Generation," or those who were aware of this incredible hippie festival held for "three days of peace and music" in August 1969 on Max Yasgur's dairy farm in upstate Bethel, New York, may recall announcer Chip Monck's cautionary words about the "brown acid":

> *"To get back to the warning that I've received, you might take it with however many grains of salt you wish, that the brown acid that is circulating around us is not specifically too good. It's suggested that you do stay away from that. Of course, it's your own trip, so be my guest. But be advised that there is a warning on that, okay?"*

This has to rank among the most magnificent public service announcements of all time. I'm not sure how accurate Monck's warnings were, or what effect they had, but that is beside the point. Because, fast forward six decades, and it's pretty clear that the acid is still floating around – in whatever form and color – and it's finding a legitimate place in the armamentarium of psychiatric treatment.

I did not attend Woodstock. I was in high school at the time and too young to appreciate the significance of events that were about to unfold. (Could anyone really anticipate the magnitude of the event?) However, I have seen the full-length feature film a number of times, and I suppose that this counts me as an expert of sorts.

Mike Greenblatt, author of *Woodstock 50th Anniversary: Back to Yasgur's Farm,* wrote that when he returned home from the festival, his mother clutched him to her bosom and cried. "Since then," he says, "I've done nothing my entire life but listen to music and tell people about it [Woodstock]."

There were at least 400,000 other stories from those who made it to Woodstock, and millions more from people who wished they were there but never made it. Maya Angelou said: "There is no greater agony than bearing an untold story inside you."

The reason I wrote this piece was to let you know that the brown acid at Woodstock and the new-found popularity of psychedelic drugs in psychiatry are not the headlines. No. The reason I wrote this essay was to remind you that the real story behind Woodstock is the untold stories that never saw the light of day. Let's not forget to honor our patients by telling their stories and sharing ours with them.

17.
Our Secret Life Comes Out in Prose and Poetry

"Don't get it right, just get it written."
— James Thurber

I was having an online discussion with my narrative medicine instructor and a classmate (a physician) via the secure messaging app WhatsApp. I brought up the subject of "forgiveness," and our instructor broached the topic of relationships, specifically the one between herself and her older sister, which she described as "stressed."

I understand very well the harm that can be inflicted in sibling relationships. My older brother tortured me. The great poet Jimmy Santiago Baca, who first came to write poetry as a young man in prison, wrote: "Being a human being without forgiveness is like being a guitarist without fingers or being the diva without a tongue." I have forgiven my brother. Now in our 70s, we are best friends. I did not sense that type of bond existed between my teacher and her sister.

My classmate referenced James Thurber's "The Whip-Poor-Will," a short story printed August 9, 1941 in *The New Yorker*. My classmate said it was a story of "blame and forgiveness," although in reality it's a very sordid tale: the song of a whippoorwill drives a man to murder his wife and two servants and kill himself.

My classmate went on, "James Thurber had one of his eyes damaged by an arrow from his brother while playing [the game] William Tell. His brother missed the apple on James' head! Years later Thurber wrote 'The Whip-poorwill.' I wrote a thesis about this story as an undergrad, and I missed the connection that his brother's name was William (whip-poor-will!)."

My classmate then messaged our instructor: "Maybe story/poetry has a place in your sister's life. Or maybe you could ask her about it [forgiveness] in poetry?"

I felt compelled to protect our instructor from a possible swell of emotions, so I quickly change the subject and commented, "Thurber created Walter Mitty," alluding to "The Secret Life of Walter Mitty," a 1939 short story centering around Mitty's daydreams as a wartime pilot, a brilliant surgeon, an assassin, and a fearless soldier. (Mitty escapes his mundane existence through his vivid and adventurous imaginations.) I ended our three-way dialog by texting, "our secret life comes out in prose and poetry," and our instructor endorsed my comment with a heart emoji, without any further mention of "forgiveness."

Our secret life does indeed manifest in prose and poetry. Writing is a form of expression that allows us to explore and communicate our innermost thoughts, feelings, and experiences, including those we might not openly share in our everyday lives.

Walter Mitty's flights of fancy have several implications for doctors, even if physicians are not writers. First, it highlights the importance of imagination in the medical field. Often, medical professionals are so focused on the technicalities and details of their work that they forget the power of creativity and imagination. This story serves as a reminder that medicine is not just a science; it's an art that requires creativity and out-of-the-box thinking (see essay 32).

Secondly, the story emphasizes the power of narrative in understanding patients. Walter Mitty's daydreams provide insights into his psyche, fears, and desires. Similarly, physicians should not underestimate the importance of patient narratives in understanding their experiences, emotions, and perspectives. By listening to and documenting these narratives, physicians can provide more empathetic and personalized care.

Lastly, the short story underscores the role of storytelling in medicine. The medical field is filled with stories – of diseases, treatments, successes, and failures. By effectively telling these stories, physicians can educate others, drive change, and contribute to the advancement of medicine.

"The Secret Life of Walter Mitty" serves as a reminder for all physicians to value imagination, patient narratives, and storytelling in their practice. For physician writers, especially, our secret lives can be further understood and shared through prose and poetry and also evolve and transform through the act of writing. Using this essay as an example, what began with a conversation about forgiveness morphed into a narrative about self-expression, quite by accident, based on a literary prompt, i.e., Walter Mitty.

Make no mistake, prose is a powerful medium to explore our secret selves. Through detailed narratives, character development, and plot, we can express our hidden desires, fears, and dreams. Prose allows us to create scenarios where we can live out these secret lives, much like Walter Mitty does in his daydreams. These narratives can be cathartic, allowing us to confront and understand our inner selves better.

Poetry, with its emphasis on emotions and imagery, can provide a more abstract and symbolic representation of our secret lives. It allows us to express our deepest emotions and thoughts in a condensed and potent form. Metaphors, similes, and other poetic devices enable us to hint at our hidden selves without explicitly stating them.

Whether through pose or poetry, the act of writing can serve as a form of self-discovery and introspection, helping us uncover our unique and hidden identities. Thurber commented: "The original of Walter Mitty is every other man I have ever known. When the story was printed in *The New Yorker*...six men from around the country, including a Des Moines dentist, wrote and asked me how I had got to know them so well. No writer can ever put his finger on the exact inspiration of any character in fiction that is worthwhile, in my estimation. Even those commonly supposed to be taken from real characters rarely show much similarity in the end."

Thurber's observation is a testament to our individuality, a distinctiveness that transcends our occupation and status in life. At the same time, all humans share similar bonds in their thinking and capacity to imagine, probably because storytelling is hardwired into our brains to some extent. Film critic David Fear wrote, "Whatever the inspiration, a huge part of what makes the short story so resonant for us card-carrying members of the Daydream Nation is the way its style replicates our mind-set so accurately, dipping in and out of absurdist imaginary situations with an admirable agility."

If you're the type of person that is on the introverted side, like me, and concerned about how individuals may view you for speaking out or simply for being yourself, consider writing as an alternate way to express your authenticity and inner self. And, if you are a physician, you would do well to remember that your day-to-day experiences and interactions with patients, families, caregivers, and others connected to health care are considerably fuller and more exciting than Mitty's real life as a nebbish conscripted into chauffeuring his wife on Sunday errands.

Thurber's tragic childhood accident resulted in a condition known as sympathetic ophthalmia, and it almost blinded him. He admitted that writing "Whip-Poor-Will revealed his anger toward five unsuccessful eye operations. Thurber's near-blindness caused him to grow up to see the world in a bizarre and hilarious light, blurring the line between fantasy and reality in his works (see essay 37). However, you don't have to resort to fantasy and grandiose delusions to get by in life. Write about your encounters, don't envision them. You *are* living the dream!

18.
Reflections on Human Suffering

Searching for a silver lining in depression.

I was in my upstairs office when I heard the doorbell ring. I ran downstairs to open the door, unable to see through the opaque window who was on the other side. I opened the door and there stood an elderly Black man and woman, well dressed, with leaflets and literature. I immediately recognized that this was an unsolicited proselytization.

"Can I help you," I inquired? The woman handed me a pamphlet and asked, "Do you believe that human suffering will end?" I glanced at the pamphlet but not really searching for the answer.

"I'm tied up at the moment ma'am, but 'no,' I do not believe suffering will end." I returned the pamphlet, thanked her, and closed the door." I was borderline rude. I was pressed for time.

I might have answered "yes" to her question at one time, that human suffering will end one day, but how could I answer in the affirmative now, less than three weeks after the unthinkable loss of life of defenseless Israelis at the hands of Hamas terrorists. Carnage was the predominant image in my mind when I answered "no" as to whether human suffering will ever end.

The two individuals at my front door were Jehovah's Witnesses. There is no doubt they would beg to differ with me. Jehovah's Witnesses believe the end of suffering is at hand, and God has promised to do away with all causes of human suffering, including crime, warfare, sickness, and natural disasters. I wasn't in the mood to debate them, although had I been, I might have chosen to debate "sickness" rather than "warfare." Each is equally deserving as a discussion point, but I'm a healer and not a politician.

I wanted to tell my impromptu guests that as a physician, I am committed to alleviating human suffering to the best of my ability through medical science and compassionate care. However, it is important to understand that suffering, in its various forms, is a part of the human condition. It is influenced by a multitude of factors beyond physical health, including psychological, social, and environmental factors.

While medical advancements continue to improve our ability to treat and prevent diseases, thus reducing physical suffering, it is beyond the scope of medicine to completely eliminate all forms of human suffering. This is because suffering is not just biological but also psychological, emotional, and existential.

However, this doesn't mean we should stop striving to alleviate suffering wherever we can. As physicians, we are tasked with not only treating illness but also improving quality of life, providing comfort, and offering psychological and emotional support. These efforts, both big and small, contribute to reducing suffering in the world.

It's also been said that suffering can sometimes lead to personal growth and resilience. Many philosophical and spiritual traditions argue that suffering is a necessary part of life and can lead to greater wisdom and empathy. As a psychiatrist, I don't fully agree with that reasoning, especially as someone who has suffered in the past from serious depression. I would not wish it upon anyone.

Sir Winston Churchill was plagued throughout his life from recurrent episodes of severe depression, which he ruefully characterized as his "black dog," a faithful companion, sometimes out of sight, but always returning.

According to the *Oxford English Dictionary*, the first use of the phrase "black dog" to describe melancholy and depression was in 1776 by Dr. Samuel Johnson, the creator of the *English Dictionary*, who suffered from clinical depression. Johnson called his melancholia "the black dog" in conversations and correspondence with his friends. Andrew Solomon, in *The Noonday Demon: An Anatomy of Depression*, states that both Abraham Lincoln and Winston Churchill "suffered from depression [and used] their anxiety and their concern as the basis for their leadership."

I find it difficult to believe that severely depressed persons can be effective leaders given that severe depression results in marked indecisiveness, apathy, complete loss of pleasure (anhedonia) and slowed down mental and physical activities to the point of paralysis (psychomotor retardation). All of these features hamper the ability to lead.

William Styron, author of *Sophie's Choice*, said: "The pain of severe depression is quite unimaginable to those who have not suffered it, and it kills in many instances because its anguish can no longer be borne." Styron's memoir, *Darkness Visible*, discusses his public fight with depression, and his advocacy has helped others who have struggled with mental illness. Unlike another book I have read, *The Secret Strength of Depression*, depression has no silver lining in my opinion. We are not better for having survived it. In fact, we are more likely to experience it again.

The late *60 Minutes* host Mike Wallace was also very public about his battle with depression and suicide (overdose). He had difficulty eating, sleeping and concentrating, and even after revealing to a family physician that he was worried about his mental state, Wallace said the doctor told him, "You're a tough guy. You'll get through it." Wallace's wife Mary believed he was suffering from clinical depression, but the doctor reportedly told the couple, "Forget the word 'depression' because that'll be bad for your image."

Had Wallace been successful in completing suicide, what would his image have been then? His body would have been six feet underground, and his legacy would have been tarnished due to the stigma of depression and suicide. Fortunately, Wallace sought psychiatric treatment and regained his health through psychotherapy and antidepressant medication.

I've witnessed too much suffering in my career – from sickness and mental illness alone, let alone other types of suffering mentioned by the Jehovah's Witnesses. My lived experience as a physician would have been the basis of informing them that I believe it's unlikely that human suffering will ever completely cease. However, I would have added that it is our duty as physicians, and as members of society, to work tirelessly to alleviate suffering as much as possible, and in the words of William K. Root, MD, "be worthy to serve the suffering."

19.
The Medical Establishment's Fight for and Against Diversity

Improving the practice of medicine through non-discriminatory, bridging ideologies.

The ruling of the Supreme Court of the United States (SCOTUS) to eliminate race-conscious decision-making from college admissions was openly challenged by the medical establishment. The American Association of American Medical Colleges (AAMC), the Medical Board of California, and the John A. Burns School of Medicine (JABSOM) at the University of Hawaii (among others) vowed to continue their efforts to diversify education and medical staffing despite the Supreme Court's prohibition against the use of race and ethnicity in admissions decisions.

The AAMC was quick to act and step into the ring. On June 29, 2023, the same day SCOTUS reversed long-standing affirmative action admission policies at Harvard and the University of North Carolina, the AAMC said they were "deeply disappointed" with the Supreme' Court's verdict, writing, in part: "We remain committed to enhancing health professional education and practice by emphasizing critical thinking, innovation, effective communication with all patients, and increased access to patient care for an increasingly diverse population … We will work together to adapt following today's court decision without compromising these goals. The health of everyone depends on it."

The Federation of State Medical Boards (FSMB), which considers itself the "voice" for state medical boards, actually began addressing diversity, equity, and inclusion initiatives before SCOTUS weighed in. The FSMB formed a task force in 2021 to "address systemic racism, implicit bias, health equity in medical regulation and patient care." Legislation soon followed in California that mandated "continuing education courses … that includes the understanding of implicit bias [defined as] the attitudes or internalized stereotypes that affect our perceptions, actions, and decisions in an unconscious manner … and often contributes to unequal treatment of people based on race, ethnicity, gender identity, sexual orientation, age, disability, and other characteristics."

Individual medical schools also entered the fray. The John A. Burns School of Medicine (JABSOM) at the University of Hawaii issued a Statement on SCOTUS Race-Conscious Admissions Ruling affirming that they will not be deterred from their many diversity initiatives and programs encapsulated in their vision, mission, and values. JABSOM embraces diversity and inclusion as part of their shared Hawaiian, Asian, and Pacific values, promoting the recruitment and retention of students, faculty, and staff, who are representative of the diverse population of Hawaii, where whites are in the minority.

JABSOM's goal is similar to many other medical schools, including my alma mater the Lewis Katz School of Medicine at Temple University, which incorporates community members on the admissions committee to ensure a diverse representation of students. Temple's associate dean of admissions commented: "There is a unique community in North Philadelphia. A big part of a medical student's education is providing care within this community and learning to understand the people who live in our community and the challenges they face."

Attracting and admitting minority medical students will increase the supply of minority physicians in impoverished areas. People of all races tend to prefer to see physicians who are similar to them in race or ethnicity, and when patients are of the same race as their providers, they report higher levels of satisfaction and trust and better communication and health outcomes. Race-conscious admissions seemed to have achieved their desired effect: the percentage of minorities entering medical school has increased the past several years. Not surprisingly, ananalysis of affirmative action bans in six states found that medical school enrollment of students of color who were members of underrepresented groups fell roughly 17% after the bans were instituted.

JABSOM's class size is relatively small, approximately 75 to 80 students. Its 2019 entering class enrolled 68 (88%) Hawaii and Pacific Island residents and 9 (12%) non-residents from the mainland and Canada. Ten percent of students were white. Of the total 1980 medical school applicants, the overwhelming majority – 1682 (85%) – were non-residents, giving an undisputable advantage to the residents of Hawaii and the Pacific Islands due to the high rejection rate of out-of-state students (about 50 times more likely to be denied admission).

Although *U.S. News & World Report* ranked JABSOM #16 in best medical schools for primary care, for all its student and employee diversity pipelines and partnerships, the school ranks only #80 for diversity. JABSOM doesn't even rank among the top 100 schools in most graduates practicing in rural or medically underserved areas. This sad fact is in contradistinction to the school's raison d'être, which is to train individuals from disadvantaged socioeconomic and/or educational backgrounds who ostensibly have a stronger commitment to serve in geographical areas of need. Many JABSOM graduates have moved to the mainland to practice, where they have found more attractive employment options and a lower cost of living.

Headlines other than the Hawaiian diaspora have cast diversity in a negative light. Two physicians and the conservative organization Do No Harm filed a lawsuit seeking a permanent injunction to stop the California medical board from implementing implicit bias training, claiming that an instructor cannot be compelled to "espouse the government's favored view on a controversial topic," further noting that "[e]ven assuming sufficient evidence exists that implicit bias in health care is prevalent and results in disparate treatment outcomes, there is no evidence-based consensus that trainings intended to reduce implicit bias are effective."

Do No Harm is a group of medical and policy professionals who oppose race-conscious medical school admissions and other policies that incorporate identity-based considerations into health care decision-making. According to the website of Do No Harm, the group has filed a number of lawsuits or complaints "to combat the influx of discriminatory and divisive ideologies in medicine," including a minority scholarship program in Arkansas that excludes white and Arab-American applicants, Project Hope and its Journal *Health Affairs* for excluding whites from a fellowship, Pfizer for excluding whites and Asians from its fellowship, and the Biden administration for "injecting a race ideology into medical regulations."

All this acrimony raises the concern that medicine is headed toward troubling times. It is entering an unsettling and tenuous state where every action that embraces diversity has an equal and opposite reaction, more vocal and certainly less civil than the previous one. The blowback can be seen not only in the anti-woke movement but also in ordinary citizens who feel discriminated against: more than half (55%) of white Americans said that, generally speaking, they believed there is discrimination against them today, according to a poll taken in 2017 by NPR, the Robert Wood Johnson Foundation and the Harvard T.H. Chan School of Public Health.

The survey sampled 3,453 adults; 902 were white. Interestingly, 84% of whites believed discrimination also exists against racial and ethnic minorities. Indeed, people from every racial or ethnic group surveyed said they believe theirs faces discrimination – not only whites, but African-Americans, Latinx, Native Americans and Asian-Americans.

Most notably, while a majority of whites in the poll felt discrimination against them exists, a much smaller percentage said that they have actually experienced it. The most insightful thing I can say is that discrimination is different when you experience it than when you talk or think about it. I may have grown up white and privileged in suburban United States, but whenever I visit Hawaii – at least twice a year – I quickly realize I am a minority. I wouldn't have stood a snowball's chance in hell gaining admission to JABSOM because I do not look like the population they aim to teach and serve and I do not share their same lived experiences. Nor could I count on SCOTUS anymore to bolster my chances of being admitted.

20.
How Will Tomorrow's Medical Students be Different?

New skills before and during medical school may enhance diversity and development.

The future of medical students appears promising and challenging at the same time. While there will be abundant opportunities for medical students to explore various fields of medicine, they will be challenged by high stress levels, financial burden, and unprecedented competition for prestigious residencies. How will they fare? In what ways will tomorrow's medical students be different than past generations? Here is a brief overview of what medical school applicants can expect, and how their training will provide an advantage over previous graduates, in my opinion.

A main advantage comes from training prior to matriculation into medical school. Many of the standards for acceptance into medical school by which my generation (Baby Boomers) and others were judged are no longer relevant. The soft sciences – as opposed to the hard sciences – now have standing in premedical curricula, especially courses in psychology and sociology. At Philadelphia area medical schools, for example, calculus is required at only one of eight MD or DO granting institutions (Penn State).

The Association of American Medical Colleges (AAMC) added a psychology-sociology ("psych-sosh") section to its MCAT standardized admissions exam in 2015. The revised MCAT reflects the importance of learning how to think and solve problems, with more questions requiring that future doctors use analytical skills rather than simply memorize material. Prerequisite courses in the social sciences may also yield students who are emotionally intelligent as well as clinically competent.

It's telling that in a survey of physicians trained in my era – those graduating college between 1955 and 1982 – the greatest unmet need was "skill with people," and my peers wished they had taken more courses in art, history, literature, and music while in college. Nowadays, some of those subjects are expected if students want to earn a spot in medical school, even if they reserve the right to "fall asleep in [their] seats during lectures," wrote acclaimed physician-author Chris Adrian, MD.

After decades of welcoming science nerds, medical educators have finally placed more emphasis on the humanities in medicine. Medical students need to be competent in the humanities in order to converse intelligently with a heterogeneous health-conscious public. Once accepted into medical school, students can augment their literary competence through narrative medicine programs, now offered at roughly 80% of medical schools. These programs aim to teach medical students sensitive interviewing and empathic listening skills, combined with storytelling and writing skills to acknowledge the struggles of their patients, as well as their own.

The AAMC has also created an optional exam to evaluate the "situational judgment" of students applying to medical school. The Professional Readiness Exam, formerly known as the AAMC Situational Judgment Test, consists of 30 hypothetical scenarios and 186 related questions that test the effectiveness of students' remedies to hypothetical situations encountered in the classroom and practice. The appropriateness of students' responses is a proxy for their readiness to enter medical school, as determined across eight core competencies such as service orientation, cultural competence, and teamwork.

Typical dilemmas presented to students include: (1) how to deal with a classmate who violates patient privacy on social media; (2) how to ensure a patient's cultural customs are respected in the event something unexpected occurs following surgery; (3) how to seek help when the stress of a clerkship in emergency medicine is beginning to affect sleep and judgment; (4) how to address a lecturer who is quick to dismiss multiple valid perspectives on a subject; and (5) how to deal with a classmate who has assumed a deceased immigrant was "undocumented," or a person's stomach pain was fabricated because they were homeless.

Another similar test, made by Toronto-based Acuity Insights, is called Casper. This assessment evaluates aspects of students' social intelligence and professionalism such as ethics, empathy, problem-solving, and collaboration. The evaluation offers admissions assessments that give each applicant the opportunity to showcase their attributes beyond their grades and to differentiate themselves from other applicants.

As discussed in the preceding essay, the removal of affirmative action admission policies by the Supreme Court of the U.S. (SCOTUS) has not deterred medical schools from efforts to select diverse students, deemed necessary to reduce health disparities. Conducting holistic reviews of applicants and searching for unique personal characteristics complies with the SCOTUS ruling and supports diversity. In addition, some medical schools have instituted community outreach and "pipeline" programs to attract a more diverse applicant pool. The University of California Davis School of Medicine has maintained a remarkably diverse class of students by assessing their socioeconomic status rather than their race and ethnicity (affirmative action admissions have been banned in California public colleges since 1996). A heterogeneous workforce has been shown to improve patient outcomes and increase trust in the doctor-patient relationship. Furthermore, teaching diversity, equity, and inclusion across medical school campuses fosters a sense of belonging among staff and faculty and the patients they serve.

Tomorrow's medical students will be vastly different from their predecessors not only due to their premedical training and selective screening for admission, but also due to changes in medical education methods, evolving technological advancements, and the continuously shifting healthcare landscape.

With the rise of digital health technologies such as telemedicine, artificial intelligence (AI), and machine learning, future medical students will be better technologically equipped. They will be trained in using advanced tools to diagnose, treat, and communicate with patients. In addition, improvements in virtual and augmented reality will provide students access to cutting edge learning tools. This will make their education more interactive and practical, potentially facilitating better understanding and knowledge retention.

AI in particular holds significant promise for medical students, training them to operate at a higher cognitive level and reducing time gathering data and information from multiple sources. According to Harvard Medical School educator Bernard Chang, MD, MMSc, "students ought to be able to move further along the developmental progression of reporter, interpreter, manager, and educator earlier in their training, reaching functional levels at which their cognitive talents will be most valuable in an AI-assisted clinical environment."

Future medical students will increasingly learn to work within and lead multidisciplinary teams. As the healthcare system shifts focus from treatment to prevention, medical students will pay closer attention to the social determinants of health and emphasize preventive care.

The COVID-19 pandemic has shown the importance of adaptability in healthcare. By virtue of having lived through the pandemic, medical students will show resilience and flexibility to changes in the healthcare environment, including changes in the way medicine is practiced and health systems achieve their goals. The whims of private equity and the business of medicine will become second-nature to them. With the rise of healthcare startups and new medical ventures, future medical students will learn entrepreneurial skills to innovate and improve the healthcare system. In fact, in 2022, there were 92 MD/MBA programs among 151 U.S. medical schools (60.9%). Clearly, tomorrow's medical students will be unlike any cohort of doctors in my time.

21.
The Physician of the Future May Not Practice Medicine

Doctors are looking for zebras, red herrings and rabbits.

In the previous essay, I marveled at the qualities that will set apart tomorrow's physicians from previous generations. And while everything I wrote I believed to be true, I suppose I neglected a major concern, a big blind spot as it were. In order to become clinicians, medical students must first enter practice. That seems obvious, but a recent report gives reason to pause and reflect on medical students' experiences and career trajectories.

The report, Clinician of the Future: 2023 Edition, was released by the health science and journal publisher Elsevier in October 2023. In all, 2,212 medical and nursing students from 91 countries were surveyed between April and May 2023. Findings also included two roundtable sessions with stakeholders and faculty in the U.S. and the U.K.

A quarter of aspiring physicians in the U.S. – double the percentage in the rest of the world – said they were considering quitting their studies, with many expressing concerns about their mental health and how they can find a satisfying balance between the demands of school and life.

Among the U.S. surveyed medical students, 54% said they were concerned about their mental health, 57% expressed concerns about experiencing burnout, and 65% were worried about how clinician shortages would affect them. An unrelated 2023 survey showed that medical students have higher rates of burnout than physicians and residents.

The most striking statistic, however, was that 54% of medical students globally – 61% in the U.S. – said they viewed their current studies as a stepping stone to broader careers in health care that don't involve treating patients. The main career paths students were interested in were public health management, research, and business consulting. The high percentage of students considering their studies as stepping stones to administrative and support roles was surprising, as those sorts of decisions are typically seen later in medical careers.

The question in my mind is whether the pressures of medical school are pushing students to rethink their careers, or whether there is something about these students or their education that makes nonclinical careers attractive to them? Of course, both a "push" and a "pull" could simultaneously exist, but the study did not specifically address this question. Here are some of the issues voiced by one student (see essay 45) that make him want to forgo practice:

- Hopelessness about patients' health

- Chronic conditions for which there is no cure or effective treatment

- Disappointment over the influence of insurance coverage in determining which treatments patients receive

- Frustration at the amount of documentation, which seems to take precedence over time spent with patients; and

- Discouragement by the overall health environment where it seems workers do not feel valued or happy to be there

It seems to me that students who are genuinely interested in alternatives to practicing medicine will find greater fulfilment compared with those who simply want to escape the stress or unfulfillment of future practice. Sylvie Stacey, MD, MPH, author of *50 Nonclinical Careers for Physicians* wrote, "I realized early in medical school that a conventional career in medicine wasn't right for me. I eliminated medical specialties as career options as fast as I rotated through them…Nonclinical work has continued to be satisfying and challenging since I completed medical training."

Sanjana Vig, a dual-degreed (MD/MBA) anesthesiologist, wrote: "I made the decision to get an MD/MBA when I was still in high school. I had an interest in medicine but hated the idea of being yet another Indian doctor. How unoriginal. So, when my dad introduced me to someone who had done this dual degree, it was my 'aha!' moment."

As mentioned in the prior essay, MD/MBA programs have become very popular. Over 90 medical schools in the U.S. offer the combined degree. MD/MPH programs have also become gateways to alternative careers. Timing is important. Although an extra degree can be earned in medical school, a more common pathway is to return to graduate school some-time after residency – for example, through an executive MBA program. Completion of residency and board certification are viewed as critical credentials for physicians even if they choose not to practice, so many doctors prefer to not interrupt their medical training until after they pass their professional boards.

According to Stacey, the primary career sectors available to physicians outside of practice are:

- Health Care Services Delivery

- Health Care Finance and Management

- Pharmaceuticals, Medical Devices, and Biotechnology

- Technology and Innovation

- Professional and Financial Services

- Writing and Communications

- Public Health and Government

- Education and Research

- Nonprofit Sector (e.g., advocacy groups, professional organizations, certification and accreditation)

- Consumer Health

- Consulting and Entrepreneurship

Stacey's website (https://lookforzebras.com) is a treasure-trove of information for medical professionals interested in exploring nonclinical opportunities. She has a vibrant blog and online community named *Look for Zebras*. It's an inside joke. In medical school, students are told not to look for zebras when they hear hoofbeats, meaning common conditions occur commonly, and those are the ones that should be considered first. "Looking for Zebras" is the equivalent of diagnosing a rare disorder instead of a heart attack when a patient presents acutely with crushing chest pain.

Stacey remarks on her website: "As a physician or other medical professional, there are tons of jobs out there that will leave you burned out and unfulfilled. These are horses. Zebras in your career are the rare opportunities that are truly a great fit for your interests, your personality, and your career objectives. Zebras seldom fall into your lap. You need to look for zebras."

Another expression that has a connotation similar to zebras is "red herring," as in, "it's a red herring," meaning the medical clue or information you are acting on is, or is intended to be, misleading or distracting. Don't go down that rabbit hole!

I must admit I was one of those medical students who looked for zebras early in my career. No field of medicine other than psychiatry held my interest. One day, in my senior year of medical school, while on an internal medicine rotation, I snuck off to the hospital library. The most recent edition of *The New England Journal of Medicine* lay before me. I picked it up and scanned the articles. My attention was drawn to the clinicopathological conference, a discussion about a patient with eosinophilic fasciitis (talk about zebras!). Fascinating, but not relevant to psychiatry. I read it anyway.

The next day, students and residents had gathered in a conference room to hear a lecture by a senior attending. He began to pimp us. Sure enough, he was describing the symptoms of the patient I had just read about in the journal. "What is this patient's diagnosis," the attending demanded, peering over his half-rimmed glasses, staring down the students and residents. I waited a few seconds. No one responded, so I blurted out, "eosinophilic fasciitis."

You could literally hear my classmates' and residents' jaws drop. The correct answer had come from a future psychiatrist of all people, someone who was already beginning to be ignored by his peers and deemed non-mainstream, not having the "right stuff." The attending was likewise astonished, chiding the residents rather than complimenting me for having the answer.

Despite Elsevier's survey, I'm not convinced that a high percentage of medical students will actually forsake practice. The pressures facing current students have not gone unnoticed by medical school educators, who are attempting to remedy the many problems students must overcome in medical school.

In addition, students' enthusiasm about technology and the use of artificial intelligence in education, plus their genuine passion to heal – 89% of medical and nursing students worldwide reported they were still devoted to improving patients' lives – will propel most of them into practice. The survey findings give all of us working in healthcare much to consider as we strive to give today's medical students the best chance to succeed in their medical careers.

22.
Emotional Intelligence Must Guide Artificial Intelligence

There was a reason Jean-Luc Picard was Captain of the U.S.S. Enterprise and Data was not. Make it so!

There's certainly no deficit of information regarding artificial intelligence (AI) and how it will revolutionize – or destroy – the practice of medicine. To make the implementation of AI more palatable, there is a drive to drop the "artificial" in intelligence and replace it with "augmented." Either way, AI has become a lightning rod for disagreements about the potential harms of the emerging technology.

AI encompasses several technologies, including machine learning, natural language processing, and robotics, all of which have significant applications in medical practice. AI in medical practice is revolutionizing healthcare delivery by automating routine tasks, improving diagnostic accuracy, and facilitating personalized medicine. AI algorithms can analyze vast amounts of data in seconds, enabling physicians to diagnose diseases more quickly and accurately.

In radiology, for instance, AI can identify patterns in images that may be missed by the human eye, enhancing diagnostic precision and speed. AI can also predict patient outcomes based on historical data, helping doctors make informed decisions about treatment plans. Moreover, AI can outperform humans on exams.

Common applications of AI in medical practice include:

1. **Diagnosis and Treatment**: AI algorithms can analyze complex medical data to aid in the diagnosis of diseases. Machine learning models can identify patterns in imaging data, genomic data, or electronic health records that may be too subtle for humans to detect. For instance, AI is used in radiology to detect anomalies in medical images such as X-rays, CT scans, and MRIs. AI can also help in treatment planning by predicting patient responses to various treatments based on their medical history and genetic profile.

2. **Predictive Analytics**: AI can be used to predict patient outcomes, allowing for proactive care. For example, AI can help identify patients at risk of readmission or those likely to develop complications, enabling early interventions and preventive outreach.

3. **Personalized Medicine**: AI can analyze a patient's genetic data to determine their susceptibility to certain diseases and their likely response to treatment. This can enable physicians to tailor treatments to individual patients, improving outcomes and reducing side effects.

4. **Automation of Routine Tasks**: AI can automate routine tasks such as appointment scheduling, prescription refills, and patient reminders, freeing up time for healthcare professionals to focus on patient care.

5. **Telemedicine and Remote Monitoring**: AI-powered apps and devices can monitor patients' health in real-time, alerting healthcare providers to any significant changes. This is particularly useful for managing chronic conditions such as diabetes or heart disease.

6. **Drug Discovery**: AI can speed up the drug discovery process by identifying potential drug targets and predicting the efficacy and safety of drug candidates.

7. **Education**. Medical students should be expected sooner than before to function at a higher cognitive level aided by AI-based tools. AI has been shown to perform as well or better than medical students on US Medical Licensing Examination Step questions and free-response clinical reasoning testing, and AI often gets the correct diagnosis for *New England Journal of Medicine* clinicopathological cases. (It stands to reason from the previous essay that one would never have to set foot again in a medical library.) As large language models are developed that are tuned to the medical domain specifically, the educational capabilities of AI will likely be even more impressive.

In the modern healthcare landscape, not only AI but also emotional intelligence (EI), play pivotal roles in enhancing patient care, diagnosis, treatment, and overall medical practice. While AI brings about technological advancements and efficiency, EI ensures empathetic patient interactions and effective communication.

EI is crucial for fostering empathetic patient-doctor relationships, which are fundamental to patient satisfaction and treatment adherence. Doctors with high EI can understand and manage their own emotions and those of their patients, facilitating effective communication and mutual understanding. EI is also essential for managing stressful situations, making difficult decisions, and working collaboratively within healthcare teams.

Furthermore, EI plays a significant role in ethical decision-making, as it enables physicians to consider patients' emotions and perspectives when making treatment decisions. Because EI enhances the ability to identify, understand, and manage emotions in oneself and others, it is a crucial skill set that can significantly influence the quality of patient care, physician-patient relationships, and the overall healthcare experience.

Common applications of EI in medical practice include:

1. **Enhancing Patient-Physician Relationships**: Physicians with high EI can better understand and respond to their patients' emotional states, fostering trust and rapport. This can lead to improved patient satisfaction, adherence to treatment plans, and overall health outcomes.

2. **Effective Communication**: Physicians with high EI are often better communicators. They are more adept at expressing complex medical information in a way that is empathetic and understandable to patients. This can help reduce patient anxiety and confusion, leading to better-informed treatment decisions.

3. **Teamwork and Collaboration**: In a healthcare setting, effective teamwork is crucial. Physicians with high EI can facilitate better collaboration within their teams by understanding and managing team dynamics, resolving conflicts, and fostering positive relationships among team members.

4. **Stress Management**: The medical profession is often stressful. Physicians with high EI are better equipped to recognize stress in themselves and others, and to employ effective coping strategies. This can lead to improved mental health, job satisfaction, and professional longevity.

5. **Leadership**: Physicians often find themselves in leadership roles. Those with high EI can effectively guide, inspire, and support their teams, leading to improved team performance and patient care.

While both AI and EI are crucial in medical practice, they clearly serve distinct roles. Moreover, AI is far from perfect. Findings presented at the 2023 meeting of American Society of Health-System Pharmacists showed that the AI chatbot ChatGPT provided incorrect or incomplete information when asked about drugs, and in some cases invented references to support its answers. Researchers said the AI tool is not yet accurate enough to answer consumer or pharmacist questions. Of course it's not. AI is only as smart as the people who build it.

What do you expect from a decision tree programmed by an MBA and not an actual doctor? Or a large language model that is prone to fabricate or "hallucinate" – that is, confidently generate responses without backing data? If you try to find ChatGPT's sources through PubMed or a Google search you often strike out.

The fact is the U.S. healthcare industry has a long record of problematic AI use, including establishing algorithmic racial bias in patient care. In a recent study that sought to assess ChatGPT's accuracy in providing educational information on epilepsy, ChatGPT provided correct but in-sufficient responses to 16 of 57 questions, and one response contained a mix of correct and incorrect information.

Research involving medical questions in a wide range of specialties has suggested that, despite improvements, AI should not be relied on as a sole source of medical knowledge because it lacks reliability and can be "spec-tacularly and surprisingly wrong." When put to the real test – for example, making utilization review decisions, the error rate can be as high as 90%.

It seems axiomatic that the development and deployment of any AI sys-tem would require expert human oversight to minimize patient risks and ensure that clinical discretion is part of the operating system. AI systems must be developed to manage biases effectively, ensuring that they are non-discriminatory, transparent, and respect patients' rights. Healthcare companies relying on AI technology need to input the highest-quality data and monitor the outcomes of answers to queries.

What we need is more emotional intelligence to guide artificial intelligence.

AI lacks the ability to understand and respond to human emotions, a gap filled by EI. Despite the advanced capabilities of AI, it cannot replace the human touch in medicine (see essay 36). Patients often need reassurance, empathy, and emotional support, especially when dealing with severe or chronic illnesses. These are aspects that AI, with its current capabilities, cannot offer. I'm reminded of Data on Star Trek "The Next Generation." Data is an artificially intelligent android who is capable of touch but lacks emotions. Nothing in Data's life is more important than his quest to become more human. However, when Data acquires the "emotion chip," it overloads his positronic relays and eventually the chip has to be removed. Once artificial, always artificial.

A medical educator observed: "[I]f the value that physicians of the future will bring to their AI-assisted in-person patient appointments is considered, it becomes clear that a thorough grounding in sensitive but effective history taking, personally respectful and culturally humble education and counseling, and compassionate bedside manner will be more important than ever. Artificial intelligence may be able to engineer generically empathic prose, but the much more complex verbal and nonverbal patient-physician communication that characterizes the best clinical visits will likely elude it for some time."

In essence, AI and EI are not competing elements but complementary aspects in modern medical practice. While AI brings in efficiency and precision, EI ensures empathetic care and effective communication. The ideal medical practice would leverage AI for tasks involving data analysis and prediction, while relying on EI for patient interaction and ethical decision-making, thereby ensuring quality and holistic patient care.

There was a reason Jean-Luc Picard was Captain of the U.S.S. Enterprise and Data was not.

Data had all the intelligence he ever needed in his computer-like brain and the Enterprise's massive data banks, but ultimately it was Picard's intuitive and incisive decision-making that enabled the Enterprise crew to go where no one had gone before.

23.
Medicine Has Become the McDonald's of Health Care

Sorry, you can't have it your way, not even at Burger King.

I was having a conversation with a colleague about a state-funded Medicaid managed care organization (MCO). She told me that the mental health performance measures used by the state to evaluate the MCO were all "placement and provider issues," such as the amount of time children spent sleeping on the floors of social services offices or languishing in emergency departments (EDs) before being transferred for treatment or placed into foster homes.

The performance measures used by state officials also included the number of adults waiting in hospital psych units to be transferred to state hospitals and the number of children and adults waiting at home to receive outpatient services or enhancements to current services.

"This is not how MCOs should be measured," my colleague said.

"How disgusting," I replied. "Medicine has become the McDonald's of healthcare – drive-through services, where the only thing that matters is throughput and not quality."

"To make matters worse," I continued, "politicians and lawmakers created the resource shortage in the first place by failing to recognize the mental health crisis and plan for it by allocating more dollars toward essential services. Now they blame MCOs and everyone else for the service bottleneck. If that's not a case of the pot calling the kettle black, I don't know what is. Perhaps we should all take out construction loans and build more hospitals and residential and assisted living facilities?"

I admit, this is not an original idea. Health insurers have been dabbling in the brick-and-mortar business for years and, vice versa, provider-based organizations have ventured into the world of health insurance. It's just that there is such an intense push for healthcare to be more accessible to patients, especially psychiatric patients.

After all, the lack of access to evidence-based mental healthcare is the root cause for the mental health crisis in America. We must act urgently to overcome common yet difficult barriers to treatment – geographic, financial, cultural, structural, and social (poverty, education, support networks, etc.) – and do a better job of integrating psychiatry and primary care medicine.

Perhaps we should follow McDonald's lead. McDonald's pioneered the fast-food industry and is known for its efficiency and accessibility, being available worldwide. McDonald's is also vertically integrated – meaning that the fast-food chain processes the meat itself, grows its own potatoes, and transports its own materials.

With the rise of telemedicine and retail clinics in locations like pharmacies and supermarkets, the future of medicine is already beginning to resemble the fast-food industry with "fast medicine."

The comparison of modern medicine to McDonald's illustrates many trends and issues in healthcare apart from accessibility and integration, such as the drive (no pun intended) for standardization and consumerism and the over-reliance on technology. Here are some ways in which medicine has become the "new McDonald's" of healthcare:

1. Standardization: Just as McDonald's has standardized menus and processes across its outlets, healthcare has seen a significant rise in standardized treatment protocols and guidelines. This is meant to ensure consistency and quality of care. However, critics argue that it might lead to impersonal care and overlook individual patient needs. It's no wonder rival Burger King came up with the slogan "Have it Your Way" (abandoned in 2014 and now "You Rule").

2. Drive-through approach: The pressure to see more patients in less time can lead to a fast drive-through approach in healthcare, where the focus is on quick, high-volume service rather than personalized care. This can result in rushed appointments and a lack of comprehensive care. It's not uncommon for office staff to instruct patients to wait "curbside," in the hallway, at the end of a visit for their paperwork, lab slips, and other business transactions.

3. Consumerism: Like McDonald's, healthcare has also seen a shift toward consumerism. Patients are increasingly viewed as consumers or "clients" who are told they have choices in healthcare providers and decisions. But instead of delivering care that is person-centered, the emphasis on consumerism has aided marketing by rebranding healthcare. Interstate billboards advertise hospital ED wait times, but how good is the quality?

4. Cost efficiency: Both McDonald's and modern medicine strive for cost efficiency. In healthcare, this often means a focus on reducing hospital stays, increasing use of technology, and streamlining processes. However, this drive for efficiency can sometimes compromise patient care and outcomes by neglecting education and prevention and increasing medical errors and staff burnout.

5. Dependence on technology: Just as McDonald's uses technology for order taking and processing, healthcare has become increasingly dependent on technology for patient records, diagnostics, and treatment. Soon we'll be selecting treatment options from kiosks, like keying in our choice for a Big Mac over a double cheeseburger – sorry, "super-size" is no longer available.

6. Fragmented care: Similar to how a McDonald's meal is often made up of different components prepared at different stations, healthcare can often be fragmented with different specialists treating different conditions. This can lead to issues with coordination and continuity of care. Incorrect medications due to multiple prescribers are the McDonald's equivalent of receiving a hamburger with mustard and relish when you asked for ketchup and pickles.

While fast-paced medicine has some advantages, it also poses many challenges, as above. The psychiatric sequelae of assembly-line practice are most concerning, because 15-minute "medication checks" are generally insufficient unless coupled with psychotherapy, and even then, split treatment is less than optimal. As Army psychologist John Rigg has said, "Medication doesn't fix this stuff."

In addition, the mental health system is on the brink of collapse after decades of defunding and financial diversion, causing community services to dry up. De-institutionalization was a noble experiment, but it neglected the serious and persistently mentally ill individuals who now fill our prisons and seek the warmth of sidewalk steam grates during the winter.

It's critical for policymakers to consider both the medical and mental health needs of vulnerable children and older adults and balance these with personalized, quality care. I worry about our healthcare system and the politicians tasked with deciding how to fund it when they have no direct experience working in these systems and do not appreciate the gaps in service, let alone the effects of workplace distress and violence.

To make any sense of our healthcare system, lawmakers need to experience a "Big Mac Attack." They need to have their access revoked to the drive-through lanes at McDonald's lest they continue to equate fast food with fast medicine.

24.
A Look Back at Van Morrison's Self-Absorbed Descent into COVID Lunacy

Science denial and the anti-authority "What's It Gonna Take?" album.

Van Morrison has been one of my favorite musicians for decades. However, his well-publicized anti-COVID stance was indefensible in my opinion, and unfortunately his antisocial behavior is not isolated and suggests he is troubled.

Morrison's dogged anti-establishment views surrounding the COVID-19 pandemic were literally front and center in his 2022 album, "What's It Gonna Take?" his 43rd. The artwork depicts a Cold War-era couple manipulated on a hidden puppet-master's strings, suggesting we are sheeple led by politicians and healthcare leaders whose restrictive policies during the pandemic, such as masking and limiting travel, lacked proof of concept. However, the primary basis for Morrison's unabashed conspiracy spouting and bad-faith COVID denial were the unpredictable lockdowns that prohibited him from touring for several years.

In "What's It Gonna Take," he subjected us to a "Full Force Gale" of extremist ideology, conveniently ignoring the more than 1 million deaths from COVID in the United States – many of them preventable. With song titles such as "Fighting Back is the New Normal," "Fodder for the Masses," and "Fear and Self-Loathing in Las Vegas" – the latter written when Morrison was forced to reschedule a series of concerts in the desert due to the lockdown – we were served a twisted account of one man's hateful and paranoid rants, as he attempts to deny science and truth. Morrison's version of the truth would have had us believe that self-governing institutions are intent on shutting down anyone who expressed an opinion that deviated from one that is informed by scientific data.

In trying to make his case, Morrison undermined his own agency as early as the opening song. He cynically boasted he was "Dangerous" because he "said something bad [and] was getting close to the truth." He claimed he asked for the "evidence" for over a year and it wasn't shown to him, that there was no "proof." Where was he hiding?

Morrison affirmed "I Ain't No Celebrity," knowing full well he is one of the most iconic (if not feared) rock stars on the planet. Morrison claimed he was "Not Seeking Approval," yet he eternally craves an audience. The "Damage and Recovery" he described applied equally to his own misdoings as it did to COVID fatalities.

Understanding Morrison's message was never the problem; it's obvious where he stood. Rather, it was the content of his message and the purpose behind it. Morrison neglected proven facts and helped to spread fake news. I can understand his frustration with rules and regulations making it difficult (and sometimes impossible) to perform. But Morrison brushed aside COVID sequelae as if he couldn't care or it's a plain shame. COVID disinformation spread by media figures – rock and pop stars in particular – may have well been the most egregious of all because celebrities have very close bonds with their fans, just like physicians do with their patients, except their fans number in the millions, not hundreds.

Thus, although the music and musicianship on "What's It Gonna Take" are first rate, it's all for the wrong reasons. Only a few songs were penned without prosaic rage, or were at least soft around the edges. We have to wait over 70 minutes to reach the final song, "Pretending," to glimpse the Morrison of old. He deals with demons and depression – nothing new in his repertoire – but he also speaks to a life "in ruins" – a life in which he pretends to be in the "present tense" when, in fact, he is "really miles away in a trance." I wish Morrison's devotees would treat the album as the song suggests – a hoax propagated by a con man whose reality testing is slipping away.

Any sympathy for Morrison is nullified by the realization that – and even if you side with him – this album was too self-absorbed. Morrison could have widened the aperture of his world view to address the various ways inequities manifest in medicine and society. Instead, he chose to pin everything on COVID, portraying himself as a victim, as if he were the only one affected by lockdowns. Certainly, many musicians had to put their tours on hold, yet they did not feel singled out or persecuted.

Bruce Springsteen, for example, postponed touring, remarking, "After 6 years, I'm looking forward to seeing our great and loyal fans next year. And I'm looking forward to once again sharing the stage with the legendary E Street Band. See you out there, next year [2023] – and beyond." Neil Young, who, like Morrison, seems to record everything he writes with no edit button, abided by COVID restrictions, commenting on "The Howard Stern Show" that he wouldn't be touring until we "beat" COVID-19. Well, we beat it (mostly), and Springsteen and Young are touring once again.

Perhaps "What's It Gonna Take" should have come as no surprise to anyone who has followed Morrison's career and is familiar with his body of work. He has always been grumpy and ill-tempered – the first time I saw him in concert, around 1970, he walked off the stage after 45 minutes without explanation – except now his contempt for authority figures permeates his lyrics ad nauseam. Ironically, the album is listenable only when the lyrics are ignored. One protest song would have been fine, but 15 are insufferable.

Morrison turned into a reactionary anti-lockdown advocate, and I'm not sure how history will remember him. Many of us mark time by his music; it is and always will be very important to us. But "Van the Man," the poetic champion who composed indelible hits such as "Moondance" and "Have I Told You Lately," has descended into lunacy. Even his new music is at best hyperbole: the 2023 release of "Beyond Words" is just that – 17 instrumental songs. Maybe these days the best kind of Van album *is* an instrumental one where he can't throw away the rest of his career on a feeble lie.

25.
Folie en Masse at the Capitol

Mobsters with shared delusions.

In the same vein as the previous essay, i.e., through the retrospectoscope, the January 6, 2021 insurrection is not so far behind us that a psychiatric analysis of the events couldn't hurt. Specifically, what dynamics were in play that resulted in the near-overthrow of American democracy? To answer that question, a brief French lesson is in order.

Folie en masse is a French term that literally means "mass insanity." The psychiatric condition folie en masse – and its congeners folie à deux, folie à trois, etc. – refers to the transfer and sharing of delusional ideas from one person to one or more others who have been closely associated with the principally deluded individual. The diagnosis "shared delusional disorder" was dropped in the most recent (fifth) edition of the Diagnostic and Statistical Manual of Mental Disorders (DSM), although delusional disorder, which forms the foundation of folie en masse, is still well recognized as a psychiatric diagnosis in the DSM.

The essential feature of delusional disorder is the presence of one or more delusions – fixed, false beliefs – that persist for at least one month, a criterion that Donald Trump clearly met. If Trump had been removed from office under the 25th Amendment of the Constitution on the grounds that he was "unfit" to serve as president, delusional disorder could easily have been invoked as a psychiatric diagnosis and reason to relieve him. To be sure, Trump also has a narcissistic personality disorder, but delusional disorder qualifies Trump as a psychotic individual, affirming his break with reality.

The undercurrents of the January 6, 2021 insurrection at the Capitol building are best explained in terms of mass insanity caused by the transfer and sharing of delusions between Donald Trump and his followers. Many rioters were under Trump's spell and felt "instructed" by him to rush the Capitol and somehow overturn the election results. Trump's primary delusion was a psychotic fixation on the 2020 presidential election, which he believed he won but was stolen from him due to widespread voting fraud and irregularities.

"We beat them four years ago. We surprised them. We took them by surprise and this year, they rigged an election. They rigged it like they've never rigged an election before."

The imposition of Trump's delusion on his followers manifested as a call to action and incited them to storm the Capitol on his command:

"We're going to walk down to the Capitol, and we're going to cheer on our brave senators, and congressmen and women. We're probably not going to be cheering so much for some of them because you'll never take back our country with weakness. You have to show strength, and you have to be strong."

Before Trump delivered his now infamous 74-minute speech at the "Save America" rally on the Ellipse near the White House – a defiant speech given to throngs of loyal "patriots" – Trump, his family, and senior White House members were in a jovial mood and partying in a makeshift tent equipped with monitors showing the crowds gathering around the Capitol.

Kimberly Guilfoyle, Donald Trump Junior's girlfriend, was enjoying the moment dancing to the song "Gloria" (the Laura Branigan disco-inspired version). She encouraged the crowd to "fight" for Trump. Trump, himself, used the word "fight" about a dozen times during his speech, emphasizing the need for strength and repeatedly asking the crowd to fight on his behalf. He even demonstrated how to fight using boxing motions.

"We fight like hell and if you don't fight like hell, you're not going to have a country anymore."

The crowd was highly receptive to Trump in part because they had already been fired up by Rudy Giuliani, Trump's personal lawyer (at the time), who called for "trial by combat." And Donald Trump, Jr. said "we're coming for you," targeting Republicans unsympathetic to his father's efforts to remain in office. Representative Mo Brooks of Alabama opened the rally with a fiery speech proclaiming "Today is the day American patriots start taking down names and kicking ass."

The ensuing mob violence at the Capitol was entirely predictable, perhaps premeditated. Representative Liz Cheney summarized how the events unfolded for television reporters and during the public hearings of The House select committee investigating the Jan. 6, 2021, attack on the U.S. Capitol. She said, "President Trump summoned the mob, assembled the mob, and lit the flame of this attack." But Trump dismissed Cheney just as he has dismissed and discredited many of his rivals and dissenters.

"We got to get rid of the weak congresspeople, the ones that aren't any good, the Liz Cheneys of the world, we got to get rid of them. We got to get rid of them."

The psychological groundwork for the incendiary actions of those who swarmed the Capitol was laid months to years in advance, fueled by Trump's relentless stream of fantasy and falsehoods. That's how shared delusional systems develop – not overnight, but by prolonged exposure of emotionally vulnerable people to the rants of delusional and deranged people – people who tend to be admired and revered by lost souls.

Trump's delusions were primarily grandiose in nature. They also contained themes of jealousy and persecution. And the delusions he spewed were highly contagious – his unwavering belief that he won the election was cause enough for his followers to attack the Capitol in an effort to prevent the election results from being certified.

"We have come to demand that Congress do the right thing and only count the electors who have been lawfully slated, lawfully slated."

Trump's contempt for democracy imbued hatred in his followers and created a mob mentality and platform for seditious and violent behavior. Don't think for a minute that death wasn't the end game for protestors who showed up in tactical gear with weapons, explosives and zip ties. They sought out House Speaker Nancy Pelosi and chanted "hang Mike Pence," roaming the Capitol bent on hostage-taking and murder.

"Mike Pence didn't have the courage to do what should have been done to protect our Country and our Constitution, giving States a chance to certify a corrected set of facts, not the fraudulent or inaccurate ones which they were asked to previously certify. USA demands the truth!"

History is replete with examples of collective mental disorders turned violent under the umbrella of folie en masse. Many of these occurrences are historic, such as the Salem witch trials, lynching and looting mobs, and the "Manson family" slayings.

And who can forget Jim Jones, the self-proclaimed messiah who oversaw the murder-suicide of 918 of his communal followers in the jungles of Guyana (they drank cyanide-laced Kool-Aid). The Jonestown Massacre of 1978 occurred because cult members believed in their leader and his irrational ideas – Jones promised his followers utopia, but he delivered carnage.

Trump promised law and order, but he delivered a terrorist attack. Even Al Qaeda could not succeed at destroying the Capitol building on 9/11.

What specially made the Trump insanity similar to other cases of folie en masse was the conflation of politics, religion, and ideology. A noose was erected on the West Front of the Capitol, attached to a wooden beam. A man wearing a sweatshirt reading "Camp Auschwitz" was among the violent mob, as were QAnon cultists and several notorious white supremacists. Confederate battle flags waved, as did the Proud Boys flag. Very few at the gathering wore masks to protect themselves and others against COVID-19. Some insurgents professed that Trump was an agent of God and his son, Jesus Christ.

Meanwhile, at the 30-month mark following the January 6 riot at the Capitol, 1,069 of the rioters had been arrested, with approximately 561 federal defendants receiving sentences. About 335 defendants had been sentenced to time behind bars, and roughly 119 defendants had been sentenced to a period of home detention.

Trump's failure to march with his troops to the Capitol was an ultimate act of cowardice and a path Jesus would have rejected. Leaders who orchestrate folie en masse usually walk the walk, as well as talk the talk. After provoking his supporters, Trump retreated to the White House, preferring the televised version of the insurrection.

Trump was fixated on the election rather than the safety of those inside the building. As his supporters raged a riot at the Capitol, Trump tried to call football coach turned senator Tommy Tuberville to implore him to raise objections to the electoral vote count (the call went to Utah Senator Mike Lee by mistake).

Trump even attempted to rationalize the insurrection.

"These are the things and events that happen when a sacred landslide election victory is so unceremoniously & viciously stripped away from great patriots who have been badly & unfairly treated for so long."

However, Trump was reportedly displeased with the low-class appearance of his "base" as video captured their ascent into the Capitol. As a narcissist, Trump is accustomed to associating only with beautiful people who reflect a polished image resembling himself. Who did he expect would turn out to demonstrate? Businessmen in $2,500 silk suits?

Perhaps Trump's withdrawal to the White House during the insurrection and in its aftermath was a good thing. The commonly recommended treatment for shared delusional disorder it to separate the leader from his followers. The only hope of curing individuals afflicted by Trump's madness is to permanently silence the source of the inflammatory and delusional rhetoric.

Many theories have been advanced to explain the underlying psychological vulnerability of individuals who are attracted to disturbed leaders and absorb their delusions. Its roots may lie in acts of deception. *Mundus vult decipi, ergo decipiatur*, a Latin phrase, means "The world wants to be deceived, so let it be deceived." Who would know better than the author of *The Art of the Deal*?

Another explanation, one I find more compelling, can be found in James Baldwin's classic essay, "The Fire Next Time." Baldwin writes, "I imagine one of the reasons people cling to their hates so stubbornly is because they sense, once hate is gone, they will be forced to deal with pain."

You could substitute "delusions" for "hate" and still be correct.

26.
Facing Mortality Through the Narrative

"Every man is born of many men and dies as a single one."
— Martin Heidegger

Singer-songwriter Willie Nelson is going strong in his 90s. He recounts the stories behind many of his songs in the book *Energy Follows Thought*. Disarmingly honest, Nelson discusses themes of relationships, infidelity, love, loss, friendship, life on the road, and particularly poignant at this juncture of his life: mortality.

Eight songs about death and dying comprise a section in his book labeled "Last Man Standing," which is also a song that pays homage to his cronies: "Waylon and Ray and Merle and old Harlan." Reflecting on the song, Nelson observes, "Death is a deadly subject. To take off the edge, it helps to write an up-tempo song, a song with a vibe so happy that maybe for a minute I can forget the meaning of the message."

Bruce Springsteen is about 20 years younger than Willie Nelson. Springsteen has death on his mind, too. In fact, Springsteen recorded his own version of "Last Man Standing" for his 2020 solo album "Letter to You." Springsteen's "Last Man Standing" is a tribute to George Theiss, who dated Springsteen's sister and was Springsteen's bandmate in the Castile's, one of many bands that predated the E Street Band. Springsteen became the "last man standing" from The Castiles after Theis passed away in 2018.

Although Springsteen recorded "Last Man Standing" with the E Street Band backing him on the LP, he sang it solo during their 2023 concert tour – a tour that ironically was cut short by Springsteen's own ill-health due to peptic ulcer disease. The song was played about a third of the way into each concert and introduced virtually the same way every night. Springsteen would comment to the concert-goers, "Mortality brings a clarity of thought and a purpose that you might have not previously experienced. At 15, it's all tomorrows. At 73, it's a lot of goodbyes. That's why you have to make the most of right now."

It turns out that Springsteen and Nelson are in good company. There have been dozens of men "left standing" in songs and albums, not to mention films, television episodes, and literature, especially biography. If you consider musical lyrics a type of narrative – I know I do – then the subject of mortality in its many forms (death, dying, grieving, loss, etc.) is perhaps second only to the topic of love. When it comes to mortality, narrative medicine plays a crucial role in dealing with this sensitive subject. Here's how:

1. **Facilitating Communication**: Narrative medicine provides a platform for patients to express their fears, hopes, and concerns about death. It encourages open communication between the patient, their families, and the healthcare provider. This can help alleviate anxiety and promote understanding about the dying process.

2. **Enhancing Empathy**: Through the sharing of personal stories, narrative medicine fosters empathy. Physicians who practice narrative medicine are better equipped to understand and empathize with the emotional struggles that their patients are going through when facing mortality.

3. **Personalizing Care**: Each person's experience with mortality is unique. Narrative medicine values this uniqueness and encourages personalized care. By understanding a patient's personal story and their perspective on their mortality, physicians can tailor their approach to treatment and end-of-life care.

4. **Encouraging Acceptance**: Narratives can help patients come to terms with their mortality. Telling their story allows them to confront their fears, reflect on their lives, and find acceptance in their situation.

5. **Providing Support**: Narrative medicine also recognizes the importance of providing emotional support to the families of patients. By including them in the narrative process, they can better understand what their loved one is going through, express their own feelings, and find comfort.

6. **Training Physicians**: Dealing with mortality is challenging for healthcare providers. Narrative medicine serves as a tool for training physicians to handle these difficult situations with understanding, empathy, and compassion.

7. **Seeing Beyond Death**: Some of us may feel certainty about a loved one's spirit remaining after they have died. Existential writing may facilitate grieving. This possibility is often seen in children, not only in the loss of a parent or sibling, but with regard to animals and pets after they have died. Many families believe in Rainbow Bridge, a cherished gathering place where departed pets wait for their owners and cross together into Heaven.

There are numerous classic works of literature, poetry, essays, and narratives that deal with the theme of mortality. Here are some notable ones:

Books:

1. *The Death of Ivan Ilyich* by Leo Tolstoy: This novella explores the realization and denial of mortality.

2. *Tuesdays with Morrie* by Mitch Albom: This memoir discusses life lessons, including mortality, from Albom's old college professor.

3. *Being Mortal: Medicine and What Matters in the End* by Atul Gawande: This book discusses how medicine can not only improve life but also the process of its ending.

4. *The Book of Dead Days* by Marcus Sedgwick: This novel explores death and the afterlife.

5. *Death Be Not Proud* by John Gunther: A memoir of Gunther's son who died of a brain tumor.

Poems:

1. "Because I could not stop for Death" by Emily Dickinson: This poem personifies death.

2. "Do Not Go Gentle into That Good Night" by Dylan Thomas: A plea against accepting death passively.

3. "Death Be Not Proud" by John Donne: This poem explores the theme of mortality and the powerlessness of death.

Essays:

1. "The Death of the Moth" by Virginia Woolf: An essay reflecting on life, death, and the struggle in between.

2. "On the Fear of Death" by Elisabeth Kübler-Ross: An essay discussing the fear and denial of death in modern society.

Narratives:

1. "A Very Easy Death" by Simone de Beauvoir: The narrative of Beauvoir's mother's death in a French hospital.

2. "The Fault in Our Stars" by John Green: A poignant narrative about two teenagers with cancer who grapple with love and mortality.

3. "Never Let Me Go" by Kazuo Ishiguro: This dystopian narrative explores mortality through the lives of three friends who grow up together in a seemingly idyllic English boarding school.

4. "The Immortal Life of Henrietta Lacks" by Rebecca Skloot: The narrative tells the story of Henrietta Lacks, whose cells – taken without her knowledge in 1951 – have been used in some of the most important medical breakthroughs, yet she remains virtually unknown.

Narrative medicine enhances the understanding and management of issues related to mortality. Narratives about death and dying explore the human condition, the finality of life, and the meaning or purpose of our existence. Facing mortality often brings with it a commitment to write as a pathway to healing or confronting death. Narratives are an important way to remember that we are much more than illness, and even more important, to recognize the value of the patient's story in their healthcare journey.

27.
Gaining Perspective on Health Inequities

Viewing Walt Disney and Maya Angelou through divergent lenses.

"Whistle While You Work" is a song from Walt Disney's 1937 animated film, "Snow White and the Seven Dwarfs." It is sung by Snow White as she and the forest animals clean the dwarfs' cottage, hoping to earn their hospitality.

The song's circumstances in the movie reflect Snow White's optimism and positive attitude. Despite being in a tough situation – having been sent to the forest to be killed and then stumbling upon a messy, empty cottage – she remains cheerful and makes the best out of her situation.

The meaning behind "Whistle While You Work" is a message of positivity and resourcefulness. It encourages listeners to maintain a cheerful attitude, even when faced with difficult tasks or circumstances. By whistling (or finding enjoyment) while working, the task at hand becomes more enjoyable and less burdensome. The song has since become emblematic of maintaining a positive attitude and making the best out of challenging situations.

Compare (or contrast) the Disney tune with Maya Angelou's first autobiography, *I Know Why the Caged Bird Sings*. The caged bird symbolizes the author herself and more broadly, the plight of African Americans during her lifetime. The bird sings because it yearns for freedom and uses its voice as a means of expressing its desire for liberation.

The metaphor of the caged bird reflects the limitations and restrictions Angelou and other African Americans faced due to racial discrimination and prejudice. Despite these constraints, the bird continues to sing, representing hope, resilience, and the enduring spirit to rise above adversity. The song of the bird is a protest against its confinement and a statement of its existence and individuality. The caged bird sings as a form of resistance, a call for freedom, and a testament to its indomitable spirit.

The messages in "Whistle While You Work" and *I Know Why the Caged Bird Sings* are similar. Both speak to the importance of strength, courage, faith, and positivity in overcoming hardship. Both contain messages relevant to the practice of medicine and the medical profession, although clearly neither work was intended as such.

Because "Whistle While You Work" promotes a positive attitude and resourcefulness in the face of adversity, in the context of medicine this could be interpreted as a directive for healthcare professionals to maintain a positive demeanor, even when faced with challenging situations such as difficult diagnoses, long hours, or high-stress environments. Optimism can help in improving patient care as a positive attitude can help healthcare providers to better connect with their patients and provide emotional support. Additionally, it can help in promoting mental health and well-being among healthcare providers themselves.

On the other hand, *I Know Why the Caged Bird Sings* is a poignant expression of the struggle for freedom and the longing to be heard. The caged bird, despite its circumstances, continues to sing, symbolizing resilience that can accompany enslavement. This can be related to patients who, despite dire medical circumstances, continue to hope for better health outcomes. For healthcare providers, this could serve as a reminder to listen to their patients' concerns, empathize with their struggles, and work diligently to provide the best care possible.

Whereas "Whistle While You Work" is a light-hearted song encouraging positivity and productivity, *I Know Why the Caged Bird Sings* is a profound memoir that evokes deep emotions and brings attention to the struggle for freedom and equality. In terms of implications for medicine, the former emphasizes the importance of maintaining a positive attitude, while the latter emphasizes empathy and understanding.

Both works remind healthcare professionals to be compassionate, concerned, and attentive in caring for patients, and to persevere despite misfortune and against negative odds. But the story doesn't end there. There is an elephant in the room. And that elephant is race.

Doesn't it matter that "Whistle While You Work" and *I Know Why the Caged Bird Sings* are vastly different in their origins and themes, and that the former is a fantasy byproduct of white America and the latter is emblematic of oppressed African Americans? Doesn't culture make a difference in how you interpret and apply their meanings to life, and to medical practice in particular? Taken together, "Whistle While You Work" and *I Know Why the Caged Bird Sings* can be viewed as representing sharp contrasts in societal attitudes that extend to and manifest in health inequities.

Health inequities refer to differences in health status or outcomes, or in the distribution of health resources among different population groups, arising from the social conditions in which people are born, grow, live, work, and age. Health inequities result in health disparities. Here are some examples:

1. **Racial and Ethnic Disparities**: Certain racial and ethnic groups have higher rates of certain diseases, such as African Americans having higher

rates of hypertension and diabetes, or Hispanic Americans being more likely to be uninsured.

2. **Socioeconomic Disparities**: Individuals from lower socioeconomic backgrounds often have less access to quality healthcare, resulting in poorer health outcomes. These disparities can be related to income, education level, or occupation.

3. **Gender Disparities**: Women often experience worse health outcomes than men for the same condition. Heart disease, in particular, goes unrecognized or underdiagnosed. Women are more likely to be diagnosed with certain mental health conditions, such as depression and anxiety.

4. **Geographic Disparities**: Individuals living in rural areas often have less access to healthcare services, leading to poorer health outcomes. This can be due to a lack of healthcare providers in these areas, or difficulty in accessing services due to distance or transportation issues.

5. **Disability Disparities**: Individuals with disabilities often face barriers to accessing healthcare, resulting in poorer health outcomes. This can include physical barriers, such as inaccessible healthcare facilities, as well as communication barriers.

6. **Age Disparities**: Older adults may face barriers to accessing healthcare, including physical limitations, lack of transportation, or a lack of providers who specialize in geriatric care.

7. **Sexual Orientation and Gender Identity Disparities**: LGBTQ+ individuals often face disparities in health outcomes, including higher rates of mental health issues, substance use disorders, and certain types of cancer.

8. **Health Literacy Disparities**: Individuals with lower health literacy are often less able to understand health information and make informed decisions about their health, leading to poorer health outcomes.

These are just a few examples, but health inequities and disparities can exist among many other groups as well. The key factor is that these inequities are not just about individual choices, but are also strongly influenced by social, economic, and environmental factors. Unequal treatment results in unequal outcomes. Although health inequities are unfair, they could be reduced by the right mix of government policies combined with understanding and respecting cultural differences that influence patients' health beliefs and behaviors.

Past interventions designed to reduce healthcare inequities have had shortcomings, but recent interventions show promise in addressing fundamental gaps in knowledge and translation. Some of these efforts can be found in accreditation requirements and regulation guidelines from The Joint Commission, Centers for Medicare & Medicaid Services (CMS Framework for Health Equity), and other national bodies. But these small steps do not adequately recognize the urgency to eliminate health inequities. Progress has largely been isolated and slow-moving. To reach the point of true transformation, the status quo must be challenged.

Despite Angelou's traumatic upbringing as a child – she was subjected to intolerable racism, raped at age eight, and afterwards was nearly mute for five years – her ultimate triumph in life was being able to recognize and show how individuals in all their heterogeneity differ in only minor ways, as she wrote in "Human Family." She saw the best qualities in people, their virtues as well as their imperfections, yet she ignored the worst and wrote inspiringly, confidant that "we are more alike, my friends, than we are unalike."

People's character is one thing, but their health is another matter. Medical professionals should be held to the highest standards of practice in order to detect and eradicate the many systemic issues that sustain health inequities.

28.
Sending in "Tougher Canaries" Won't Fix the Problem of Physician Well-Being

A three-pronged approach aimed at medical education, training, and practice is the solution.

Many surveys and reports have acknowledged that physicians are unwell, and their numbers have reached crisis proportion. "We aren't going to fix this problem by noting that canaries are dying in the coal mine and … sending out for tougher canaries," remarked Gary Price, MD, an attending surgeon at Yale-New Haven Hospital in Connecticut and president of the Physicians Foundation, a physician empowerment organization.

Price's remarks were actually in response to a survey of medical and nursing students I discussed in essay 20. That survey reported that students were exposed to high-stakes pressures, including the financial burden of school, their first exposure to the clinical setting, and the current dysfunction in those settings. By the time those students enter residency and practice, more than half will be burned out, according to various sources. However, that's where most surveys miss the mark on what to do about physician well-being: they're either silent or don't know how to fix it. I have a three-pronged approach.

The first thing to do is totally revamp medical education. We take students who want to be doctors and lock them away in study groups and libraries with endless review videos and flashcards full of useless details. Then we submerge them in "simulations" and send them into patients' hospital rooms unsupervised and without contemporaneous feedback about their interactions with patients. After they see patients, students are left alone to process their emotional experiences and any trauma associated with their visits. They are forced to wear a false bravado as they are pimped and put down by residents who, themselves, are psychologically distressed, even damaged. The system of learning is insufferable for medical students. Should we be surprised that many come out depressed, having lost interest in serving patients, and pessimistic about their future?

Next, we need to redo the system for training residents. Clinical training based on hands-on attentive care of the patient, under close supervision by very experienced clinicians, has all but evaporated. Attendings who have shied away from extensive rounding with students and residents, or have faded into the fabric of research and pharma consulting, or simply would rather be elsewhere – anywhere other than at the patient's bedside – explains why trainees fail to fully grasp the concept of doctoring and why medical care today is so disjointed, patient-unfriendly, and often riddled with errors and failed oversight. Only altruistic physicians who are dedicated to full-time academic teaching – and are fairly compensated for it – need to show up.

I'll never forget my first night on call during my junior clerkship in surgery. I was assisting a fifth-year resident in the operating room as he repaired several lacerated tendons in a young woman's hand (her "boyfriend" brandished a knife and cut her during an argument). The surgery took place roughly between 2 and 4 a.m. Several hours later, the attending arrived for morning rounds, only to discover the resident had operated without his knowledge – that is, the attending's knowledge; there was no one to pass judgment about the resident's knowledge of intricate hand surgery. The attending went berserk, scolding the resident for not being notified prior to performing the delicate procedure. The attending said he would have come in from home to assist the resident had he known. We need more of those attendings!

Finally, we need to restore pride to the medical profession. Doctors used to go into medicine for several reasons. They wanted to take care of patients because they liked people, they loved helping others, and they welcomed the challenge of making diagnoses, performing procedures and surgery, and especially, for psychiatrists, doing psychotherapy, which is now a lost art abrogated to non-medical "therapists." Physicians liked the autonomy and collegiality of medicine, and they knew they were going to make a good living at it. All this while essentially making their own hours, working on their own terms, and withstanding the challenges of – even looking forward to – being on call. What happened?

What happened was government interference, overburdening physicians with ridiculous documentation mandates and infrastructure issues, and the corporate domination of medicine forcing private physicians to be employed, among other woes of transitioning to the medical-industrial complex. This took away physician's autonomy and their earned status to the point of simply being another hospital employee or employee of a large health system. This caused physicians to not just be responsible to patients but to corporate entities and the government. This total conflict of interest places physicians between medicine and management, where they do not belong (see the next essay). There is no reason to treat smart, ambitious doctors this way. (Jerry, I hear you singing: "Don't wanna be treated this a way …")

On top of treating doctors shabbily and with disrespect, physicians were forced to accept increasing liability and were expected to perform with perfection, so that now huge malpractice settlements deter organizations from hiring doctors – and God forbid lawyers should let physicians apologize to patients and families for mistakes. Also, continued cuts in Medicare and other health insurer's fees signaled that physicians were not valued. It all seems so surrealistic – a bad nightmare and no longer worth the price of admission to practice. Many physicians are leaving the profession in droves, and scores intend to exit over the next several years. Why should anyone be surprised that 25% of medical students intend to use medical school as a stepping stone within – or outside of – medicine rather than practice it?

Virtually everything I've read when it comes to medical students, residents, and physicians attaining well-being puts the problem squarely on them, holding doctors accountable for making the necessary changes – for example, ensuring work-life balance; encouraging healthy eating and regular exercise; practicing mindfulness; implementing regular work breaks and resilience programs; building a supportive culture; regularly assessing well-being, etc. We're too frigging busy to "build" anything. There is nothing "regular" about the practice of medicine that we should take for granted. I want to gag myself with a spoon every time I read this crap.

I see the same BS in articles suggesting structural solutions to making physicians well again, such as changing workloads and schedules; streamlining administrative tasks; enhancing team-based care; addressing financial pressures; improving workplace culture; and advocating for policy changes. Who's going to do that? Politicians and lawmakers? Hospital MBAs? They're the reason we're in this mess! Measuring physician "burnout" and holding health systems accountable for reducing its incidence is a somewhat novel idea, but let's face it, the only thing health systems are really accountable for are their bottom lines and those who back their equity.

It's time to end the rhetoric and stop pretending that coaching and coddling physicians will make them better. Broken physicians won't get fixed by sending in tougher canaries. Broken physicians may get better by breathing in fresher air.

This profession we call medicine is a sailing ship to the Devil's Triangle. Unless a course correction is imminent, unless we right the ship, there will be no more canaries to send in.

Send in the clowns.

29.
Physician Executives: Trapped Between Medicine and Management

"Turncoat" is an appropriate term for some physicians.

Many people wonder how physicians who work for health insurance companies are empowered to deny requested procedures and treatment and can do so much damage to patients yet not be accountable for their malfeasance. The term "turncoat physician" is apropos for physicians who have joined the dark side and neglected – even retaliated against – their practicing colleagues and, in the process of becoming acculturated to corporate life, have become desensitized to the plight of patients. This may apply to physicians working in government and public health agencies as well as corporations.

The modern-day equivalent of a turncoat in medicine is a doctor who exchanges the white coat for a business suit. Increasing numbers of physicians are finding private practice difficult or uncongenial and are turning to administrative opportunities as an alternative (refer to essay 21). However, caught between the desire to help patients and responsibilities to manage costs, physician executives deal with conflicting expectations. Moreover, the influence of physicians in health systems has limits, creating tension as they try to exert their authority in a sea of nonmedical executives.

Given that physicians appear to have a bright future in the corporate world, it is only natural to ask why some would turn against their colleagues in the trenches and act with indifference or disdain. Dr. Diana Chapman Walsh, an expert in public health and social behavior, attributes such behavior to the "man-in-the-middle" syndrome. In *Corporate Physicians: Between Medicine and Management*, Dr. Walsh analyzed in depth what happens to medical care when medicine is practiced by an individual who is both a physician and corporate officer. She wrote: "Company physicians have been medicine's man-in-the-middle, like the shop foreman whose misfortune it is to owe allegiance to bosses above and workers below. Foremen find ways to adapt or manipulate their situations; corporate physicians do too. But lacking predictable rules of role, company physicians have to work at the accommodation: seldom is it as straightforward for them as it is for private physicians, whose primary obligation to their patients seems relatively clear-cut."

From a psychological perspective, one may infer that, unconsciously, identification with the aggressor plays a role in shaping the "rules of the road." This defense mechanism turns victims of aggression or harm into acting like the aggressor. Identification with the aggressor is central to the Stockholm syndrome, in which kidnapping victims establish an emotional bond with their captor and take on their cause. Corporate physicians (the victims) may develop favorable feelings and behaviors toward the aggressor (the organization), and negative attitudes towards practicing physicians who are not aligned with the organizations' goals and objectives. This may explain, in part, why corporate physicians not only deny health insurance claims but also behave rudely, disrespectfully, or arrogantly toward their practicing colleagues.

Family practitioner and medical educator Dr. Sanaz Majd provides further insight into the behavior of physicians. She opines that rude, stoic, and cold behavior may develop in some physicians in order to cope with the daily practice of medicine, the so-called "detached doctor phenomenon." Majd writes: "Sometimes, it's necessary for physicians to build a concrete wall to guard their emotions. Otherwise, it would be challenging to function through our day-to-day lives as healers. Because, truly, after seeing a sick patient after sick patient, if you allow yourself to feel too much, it can significantly wear you down and render you dysfunctional."

The process of becoming detached from patients begins as early as the first year of medical school, when students must dissect a human cadaver. In conversations with medical students, Majd found that a few did reveal their emotional struggles (whether it was spiritual, religious, or personal) during gross anatomy lab. However, when the instructor asked the students, "How are you all emotionally dealing with dissecting a cadaver?" none of them spoke about their thoughts and unsettling feelings provoked by the corpse in front of them. Only "very talented and socially adept physicians learn to balance compassion with emotional detachment," according to Majd.

Research has shown that later in medical school, in the third year, the ability of medical students to empathize with patients sharply declines. This is precisely the time when empathy is most essential, because students are freed from the classroom to embark on their clinical rotations and become involved with patients. Many students never regain their empathy as their education and training progress – they are confronted with a perfect storm of factors leading to burnout: excessive workloads; long working hours; night and weekend call; comprehensive documentation requirements in EMRs; and time spent at home on work-related matters. Burned-out physicians possess negative, cynical, and hostile attitudes – not only toward patients, but also toward colleagues, treating them as objects rather than human beings.

Practicing defensive medicine to reduce the risk of malpractice litigation further erodes empathy and contributes to emotional detachment. Trainees and physicians are afraid of being sued for malpractice. Every patient could be viewed as a potential adversary. So obviously, the physician becomes a detached figure rather than an attached healer. Studies that have measured empathy, however, have shown that higher scores correlate with better patient satisfaction and outcomes. Why not measure the empathy scores of physician executives or, for that matter, medical school applicants? Medical schools could choose applicants based on both their academic performance and their potential to become caring physicians, as indicted by their empathy scores.

The answer to the question "Why do physicians turn against other physicians?" is complex and, ironically, has its roots in the medical profession itself – education, training, and practice. To cope with the vicissitudes of medical school, students become detached and less empathetic. Residents and early-career physicians have a high likelihood of developing burnout, and they begin practicing defensively, which also increases their detachment from patients. Subsequently, in mid-career, physicians may feel trapped between medicine and management, harboring anger and cynicism, culminating in behavior that is offensive and retaliatory to their peers.

I have worked both sides of the aisle in my 40-year career – my time has been divided equally between practicing psychiatry and working in industry. I have prided myself on being a physician leader who understands the business of healthcare yet has always focused on the medical foundation and tenets of care. Perhaps the kindest words a physician ever uttered were that I was a "double agent" – not a turncoat – because he recognized that, despite the fact I was an insider, I always had patients' best interests in mind. To be sure, there are physician executives who stray from that course and act punitively toward patients and their colleagues. I pray the bad actors are made accountable for the treatments they deny, especially if they stand to gain from their actions.

30.
Physicians Can Impact Marketing Through Leadership

"The medium is the message"
– Marshall McLuhan

A cartoon shows two scientists reviewing laboratory data and appearing very smug. They are content with their results and themselves. The caption reads: "One thing I'll say for us – we never stooped to popularizing science."

I've always taken an opposite approach. I have assumed that reviewing research data and disease-related information intended for promotion to doctors and patients is a good thing. Who else but physicians are best qualified to review the material for medical accuracy, completeness and realism, ensuring that all communications are scientifically credible and clinically relevant.

As a former medical reviewer in the pharmaceutical industry, I was determined to "get it right" because the information provided to physicians and patients affects the quality of care. The pharmaceutical industry also faces unprecedented challenges – not only increased government scrutiny on marketing activities – but also increased transparency demanded in clinical trials and publications.

Pharmaceutical companies spend billions of dollars to market their products, more money than they invest in R&D. Television advertising takes up the bulk of expenditures. John Wanamaker, the father of modern retailing, said, "Half the money I spend on advertising is wasted; the trouble is I don't know which half." I'd like to think that if Wanamaker had confined his efforts to pharmaceutical promotion, business savvy physicians with a keen interest in marketing would have solved his dilemma.

Physician leaders who specialize in medical marketing – a rather broad term applied not only to pharmaceutical promotion but also many other forms of medical communications – possess certain qualities that make them highly effective.

First and foremost, these physicians have strong clinical and scientific skills coupled with training or familiarity with marketing, perhaps from courses in college or business school. (A colleague of mine, the chief medical officer of a digital medical marketing company, has a master's of fine arts degree in television production and filmmaking.)

Marketing-oriented physicians have an eye for detail. They function well in teams, where they are capable of integrating multiple perspectives into a cohesive message. They frequently contribute to the creative aspects of advertising.

Russian author and physician Anton Chekhov commented, "An artist's flair is sometimes worth a scientist's brains." There is no doubt that Chekhov's medical training and practice fueled his creativity and helped him become a great playwright and author of short stories.

Physicians involved in marketing initiatives must be ethically grounded, "pushing back" when it appears that selling messages cannot be scientifically supported. Physicians must work within the parameters imposed on them by the Food and Drug Administration (FDA) and other regulatory authorities, and ensure that the interests of patients are paramount in discussions.

The FDA governs promotional activities of prescription drugs in the United States (the FTC regulates the promotion of over-the-counter drugs). When it comes to prescription drugs, pharmaceutical companies can run afoul of the FDA in several categories. The most common infractions involve:

- Promoting a drug off-label or attempting to broaden the indication of the drug.

- Making unsubstantiated claims about the drug's effectiveness or its superiority to other products.

- Omitting or minimizing important safety information and risks.

- Promoting statements about the drug's ability to improve a patient's quality of life in the absence of sufficient evidence.

The FDA operates on a risk-based approach to enforcement, meaning the agency considers primarily the impact of advertising on public health and safety. Promotional items receiving the greatest attention include newly approved products, products with significant health risks, products cited for violations in the past, products with far reaching advertising campaigns, and products cited in complaints. Direct-to-consumer marketing has become one of the most highly scrutinized areas of pharmaceutical promotion.

A risk-based approach to enforcement is necessary because the branch of the FDA that regulates prescription drug advertising – the Office of Prescription Drug Promotion (OPDP) – cannot possibly review every marketing item submitted by every drug company, even though drug companies are required to make such submissions. So, in 2010, the FDA began to enlist health care providers to help detect and report misleading drug ads. The so-called "Bad Ad Program" administered by OPDP:

- Encourages health care providers (HCPs) to be aware of the many advertisements and promotions they view every day.

- Educates HCPs explicitly about types of FDA violations seen in promotion.

- Encourages HCPs to report activities and sales and marketing messages considered false and misleading by submitting potential violations by phone, e-mail, fax, or in writing to the FDA.

- Resulted in serious enforcement actions (warning letters) to five pharmaceutical companies in the first year of operation.

Physicians have a golden opportunity to improve the quality of pharmaceutical advertising and promotion, whether working as pharmaceutical executives or surrogates for the FDA while in practice. To do so, they must be aware of the essential principles of drug promotion, which are:

- Remain consistent with the prescribing information contained in the drug's FDA-approved label.

- Give equal prominence to the risks and benefits of the drug to achieve a fair and balanced presentation.

- Be truthful and do not be misleading.

- Support all promotional claims with substantial evidence, which, in most cases will require positive results from two adequate and well-controlled clinical trials. (The standard for promoting health care economic information is competent and reliable scientific evidence directly related to a labeled indication.)

Physicians must possess a thorough understanding of biostatistics and clinical trials design and interpretation if they wish to pursue a career in pharmaceutical marketing or simply educate their patients and the public about new research findings. Imprecise terms (e.g., "large," "small," "rapid," "potent," "well-designed," etc.) should be avoided in promotion. Also, terms considered "buzzwords" by the FDA should generally be avoided in favor of more precise language. Buzzwords include terms such as "drug of choice," "gold standard," "novel," "breakthrough," "unique," "preferred," "targeted," and "well-tolerated." Terms that are highly conjecturable can be considered false or misleading.

Above all, science must rule medical marketing communications. All information must be medically accurate and verified by primary references to clinical trials or the medical literature. Speculation and opinion should be avoided, as should the use of adjectives that embellish or exaggerate marketing claims and messages. The "King's English" should prevail in all instances. Physicians working in marketing need to be good editors as they are more likely to edit advertising copy than write it.

Physician leaders working in healthcare delivery systems could certainly help portray their organizations more favorably if they step forward to join marketing teams. Creating medically responsible advertising messages is an ideal way to impact large numbers of patients, a goal all physician leaders seem to have in common. Physician leaders can help improve their company's marketing efforts by providing medical and scientific review of promotional material before it reaches the market, improving accuracy and relevance for physicians and patients. The strategic use of physicians in advertising and promotion provides medical, therapeutic and disease expertise, which may enhance the creative process, reduce medical errors, improve the quality of promotional material, and most importantly, improve the quality of patient care.

It should be obvious why physicians should stoop to popularizing medicine – because advances made in the lab cannot benefit people without actions taken outside the lab.

31.
I was Traumatized by a Patient I Never Met

Excise the skeletons in your closet by writing about them.

Soon after midnight, after a busy day on the inpatient psych unit, I slipped into a deep sleep. Then the phone rang in the residents' on-call room.

"Dr. Lazarus," the voice on the other end inquired?

"Yes," I replied, half asleep.

"This is Dr. Hendricks (not her real name) in the ER. Are you the on-call psych resident tonight?"

"I am," I answered drowsily.

Every physician knows that nightly awakenings are part and parcel of being on-call. And like most residents, I had learned how to short-circuit several stages of sleep to quickly attain alertness when paged. But tonight, it was really difficult to wake up.

"We have a patient down here. I don't think you need to see him, but I'd like to run the history by you and see if you agree with the treatment plan before we send him on his way."

I sat up in bed and said, "Sure. Go ahead."

"The patient is in his twenties. He has a diagnosis of schizophrenia, and he lives in a local boarding home. One of the staffers escorted him to the ER. The patient tells me he is hearing voices, but the voices are not telling him to do anything bad or hurt himself. Do you think it's okay to increase the dose of his Haldol from 15 to 20 mg a day and set him up with an outpatient appointment in the psych clinic?"

"Yeah, that sounds fine to me," I replied, still groggy. There were other aspects of the history that should have been explored, so I added, "Do you want me to come down and see him?"

"Oh, no. That won't be necessary," remarked the medical resident. "He looks pretty good. I'm just not too familiar with Haldol, and I want to know if bumping up his dose by 5 mg is appropriate."

"It could go higher," I explained, "but that can be evaluated further when he is seen in clinic."

"Okay, then, Dr. Lazarus. Thanks for your help."

"Is it quiet tonight?" I asked before hanging up. That was code for asking whether any other psych cases were pending and whether I could count on a good night's sleep.

"Not much happening," the resident replied. "Thanks again."

It took me less than 10 minutes to reverse the sleep cycle. I nodded off with a good feeling, comfortable that I was able to provide consultation without having to see the patient. It's about time I caught a break, I thought, given that it was spring and I was two-thirds of the way through my first year of residency.

The emergency department was run by the medical house staff, who liberally called upon psych residents to see depressed, addicted, and psychotic patients, even though these patients were supposed to be transported and seen at the community "crisis center" located at another hospital. I felt I was fortunate to be spared a midnight consultation. I also thought it was admirable that my counterpart in internal medicine attempted to handle the case herself.

Suddenly, the phone rang at 3 a.m. I awoke faster than before. "Dr. Lazarus, this is Dr. Hendricks again from the ER. You're never going to guess what happened!"

Before I could utter a word, the resident continued in a distressed tone, "Remember the patient from the boarding home? Well, the paramedics just brought him back. He jumped out the third story window and it looks like he broke both legs. We're going to take him to X-ray now, and he'll probably need surgery. I just wanted to let you know."

All I could say was, "Okay, thanks for letting me know. I'll make sure the psych consultation team sees him in the morning."

This time, I couldn't get back to sleep. I asked myself how this could have happened. The patient was stable, according to the medical resident. He did not have command hallucinations. He was not suicidal or self-injurious. I lay awake second-guessing myself – and the resident – until daybreak. I should have seen the patient, I bemoaned, rather than take the word of a physician with less experience in my specialty.

To make matters worse, in the morning, the ER staff notified the consultation-liaison (C-L) team about the incident before I did, and a rumor had spread that I had refused to see the patient in the emergency room. Shame and guilt set in immediately, like an IV infusion. I was interrogated by the upper-year resident on the C-L service. I assured the senior resident and the attending physician of the C-L service that I had offered to go to the ER at midnight, but I was told it was unnecessary. The C-L team appeared to be satisfied with my account but not with my judgment to do a telephone consultation rather than evaluate the patient in person.

Clearly, the damage was done. The patient had sustained serious injuries. The house staff dubbed him the "jumper," and I had become infamously associated with him. No matter how many times I replayed the incident, I could not forgive myself for not seeing the patient, even though a face-to-face consultation was never requested. I berated myself, thinking I should have known better, that a bad outcome would ensue.

I became overwhelmed with anxiety. I began to dread being on-call. I tried to avoid difficult cases. I became depressed, and I had all the symptoms of PTSD. My performance suffered, and it was noted by many of the faculty.

I sought the help of a senior psychiatrist, who became my therapist. He was a kind and compassionate man who understood what I was going through. He assured me that even a modest improvement in my defenses – unconscious ways of managing conflict and strong emotion – could result in a sizable improvement in my life. But he warned me, "Art, unless you can acknowledge that a patient's fate is beyond your control, you will not survive in practice."

The truth is, I did not survive in practice. A decade later I left academia for a nonclinical career (see essay 21). Along the way, I have learned from my mistakes, and hopefully I've learned how to forgive myself and seek forgiveness from those I may have harmed. Most of all, the "jumper" impressed on me that caring for seriously ill patients, and those who have the potential to become seriously ill, can significantly impact our inner lives.

"The inner life of individual physicians should, to some extent, be brought into the outer life of physicians as a collective," remarked Dena Schulman-Green, PhD, associate professor at NYU Rory Meyers College of Nursing. In that case, writing about my experience has been long overdue.

We all have skeletons in our closets that should be excised through writing. Writing about our experiences in a narrative or storytelling format can help understand and process the events better. The goal of writing in this context is not to dwell on past mistakes, but to understand, learn from, and move beyond them.

32.
Reconsidering the Art of Medicine

"Wherever the art of medicine is loved, there is also a love of humanity."
– Hippocrates

The popular notion of post-traumatic stress disorder (PTSD) is that symptoms of the disorder, such as flashbacks, intrusive thoughts, and feeling on-guard, coincide with highly stressful and specific traumatic events, for example, wartime combat, physical violence, and natural disasters. In truth, affected individuals may be exposed directly or indirectly to the stressful event. Exposure to the stressor may involve actual or threatened death, serious injury, or sexual violence. And although symptoms of PTSD usually occur within the first three months after the trauma, their onset may be delayed by six months or longer.

PTSD is usually not considered a result of medical training, but as I described in the preceding essay, it was in my case. Studies have shown that residents and physicians suffer a high rate of PTSD due to medical practice, whether or not they treat trauma patients or patients with life-threatening conditions. Apparently, the stress of practice alone is sufficient to cause symptoms characteristic of PTSD.

PTSD has also been diagnosed in professionals exposed to repeated or extreme aversive details of traumatic events in the course of health-related work. Examples include first responders collecting human remains, police officers repeatedly exposed to details of child abuse, and mental health therapists exposed to details of their patients' traumatic experiences.

Dr. James S. Kennedy, formerly at Vanderbilt University Medical Center, stated, "The resulting feeling that physicians [with PTSD] ignore most is toxic shame…the belief that one is defective. Once in practice, patient care 'retriggers' the toxic fear, loneliness, pain, anger, and shame physicians experienced in training." Unlike healthy shame, in which the individual realizes they "did bad" and attempts to atone for it, toxic shame's message is, "I am bad," and it connotes a very different internal message. Shame is a key emotional reaction after experiences of trauma, and an emerging literature suggests that researchers have failed to recognize the influence of shame on post-trauma states.

PTSD is discussed in *What Doctors Feel: How Emotions Affect the Practice of Medicine* by Danielle Ofri, MD, PhD. Ofri, an associate professor of Medicine at New York University School of Medicine, describes the riveting story of Eva, a first-year pediatric resident who was traumatized when a senior resident instructed her to let a newborn infant die in her arms – in a supply closet of the hospital no less – because the infant was doomed to a quick death due to Potter syndrome.

Ofri commented, "Eva's residency was truly a traumatic experience in which survival was the mode of operation. And the PTSD that resulted was real…Certainly, in the breakneck pace of Eva's residency, there was barely a blip of acknowledgment for the wells of sadness that bloomed, day after day."

Ofri, herself, experienced long-lasting shame and humiliation after committing an error that nearly killed a patient. Exactly two weeks into the second year of her residency, Ofri mismanaged the insulin therapy of a patient in diabetic ketoacidosis. She was severely reprimanded by a senior resident in the presence of her intern. "I could almost feel myself dying away on the spot," Ofri remarks. "The details of my insulin error in the dingy Bellevue ER are crisply stored in the linings of my heart."

Ofri later felt compelled to write an entire book about medical mistakes: *When We Do Harm: A Doctor Confronts Medical Error.* The prompt for writing the book was not only Ofri's personal experience with medical error – "I've certainly made my share of them," she admits – but also because her editor at Beacon Press had inquired (in 2016) whether medical error was the third leading cause of death in the United States, as reported in the *British Medical Journal.*

The editor also asked Ofri whether it is true, according to the famous 1999 Institute of Medicine Report, *To Err is Human*, that nearly 100,000 people die in the U.S. due to medical misdeeds – the equivalent of about a jumbo jet's worth of patients crashing on U.S. soil every day? Ofri found that the number is probably smaller, maybe half the original estimate, but the impact of just one serious mistake can have a devastating effect on the career of any doctor.

In medical school, many of us are told to "get over" our insecurities and that we do not have time to grieve our mistakes. It is only through a "hidden curriculum" that we learn that not all patients can be saved or rescued. Over time, we realize the limits of our abilities. Recognition of what it really means to be a physician – the sense of power and powerlessness, of hope and helplessness – is both an attitude and a skill that must be acquired during training.

Still, it is legitimate to ask: Who provides physicians the necessary skills to cope with loss and despair? Who consoles us when our best turns out to be not good enough? Who teaches us how to deal with uncertainty inherent in medical practice? How do we rise above the scandal and embarrassment of making a mistake? And how do we overcome our fear of making mistakes?

I was unable to resolve these issues after my traumatic experience described in the previous essay – despite psychotherapy and support from my colleagues. Assurance that I was a good doctor was insufficient. Guidance from my mentors didn't sink in. Textbooks and self-help books seemed inadequate. I rejected advice to "get tough" with patients and, alternatively, to distance myself from them.

At least my residency director was able to open my eyes to the fact that psychiatry, like other specialties, has a mortality rate – from suicide and homicide. He said I could not predict the behavior of my patients with any more accuracy than could a lay person, much less that of a patient I had never seen. In fact, research has shown that psychiatric residents are not able to predict violent behavior in patients any better than chance.

Another faculty member pointed out that practice norms vary widely across the United States. Neither evidence from clinical trials nor clinical observation can dictate action – nor inaction – in particular circumstances. The management decision for a single patient is complex, requiring a synthesis of incomplete and imperfect information and medical knowledge. "What makes you think," the psychiatrist probed, "this decision is made with any precision in the head of a sleep deprived resident?"

The psychiatrist's comment placated me and reminded me to be less hard on myself, to view practice protocols as guides to treatment, but to also realize how our emotions, prejudice, tolerance for risk, and personal knowledge of the patient guide our clinical judgment. Black-and-white approaches to patient management miss the shades of gray in between.

"We don't see things as they are, we see things as we are," noted Anaïs Nin. We learn how to obtain and accept outcomes – good or bad – even when care decisions are made with incomplete or flawed data and even in the haze of sleepiness. We allow our "sixth sense" to interact with formal approaches to the assessment and management of patients to alert us, instinctively, to potential danger and safety concerns, to channel our gut feelings and let us know how worried we should be when patients are not responding to conventional therapy. Science and artificial intelligence are of little help when we are out on a limb beyond the limits of our ingenuity and prowess. Only the art of medicine can guide us back to solid ground.

33.
The Fine Line Between Childhood Illnesses and Munchausen Syndrome by Proxy

What the "Take Care of Maya" ruling could mean for abuse accusations.

"Fine lines" in medicine refer to situations where decisions are not clear-cut and require careful judgement. Perhaps the most tenuous of lines is the one between "real" childhood illnesses and those caused by Munchausen syndrome by proxy.

Munchausen syndrome by proxy (MSBP) was first described by British pediatrician Sir Roy Meadow in 1977. The precursor diagnosis "Munchausen syndrome" had already been well established, referring to individuals who deliberately harm themselves or feign signs and symptoms of illnesses to gain medical attention. Meadow extended the boundaries of Munchausen's syndrome to include Munchausen victims, usually children, whose mothers "by falsification, caused their children innumerable harmful hospital procedures – a sort of Munchausen syndrome by proxy," he wrote in *The Lancet.*

Munchausen syndrome by proxy, also known as factitious disorder imposed on another (FDIA), refers to a specific form of child abuse in which a caregiver, typically a parent or guardian, fabricates, exaggerates, or induces physical or psychological illness in a child. The caregiver may seek unnecessary medical attention for the child, leading to unnecessary and potentially harmful medical interventions. Although the disorder has been described mainly between mothers and daughters, it has also been observed between caregivers unrelated to their patients, as well as in other pairs.

Technically there is a difference between medical child abuse and MSBP, although the terms tend to be used synonymously. The key difference lies in the motivation of the caregiver: in MSBP, the caregiver's actions are driven by a psychological need for attention or sympathy, as in classic Munchausen's syndrome, whereas in other forms of medical child abuse, the motivations can vary. So, while all cases of MSBP are considered medical child abuse, not all cases of medical child abuse are MSBP.

There are several clues to diagnosing MSBP:

- Problems that are unexplainable, persistent, or resistant to interventions that "should" work, after adequate evaluation and treatment attempts

- Serious discrepancies among the history, clinical findings, and patient's general presentation

- A working diagnosis of a disorder so rare that maltreatment is more likely

- Symptoms and signs that occur only in association with one person and/or schedule (e.g., weekly, monthly) or in the absence of a family member (e.g., whenever one parent goes on a business trip)

- A caregiver who reports that records are missing or who insists on hand carrying them without adequate reason

- Families in which other members have had problems similar to the patient's presenting problem, without adequate explanation

- A caregiver who habitually relates dramatic, exaggerated, or improbable events in relation to themselves or others

- A caregiver with previous medical or nursing experience, an extensive history of illness, or a history of factitious disorder

- Several members of the treatment team are perplexed and question the genuineness of the symptoms

The last point – suspicions among pediatric hospital treatment teams – cannot be understated. Verification of suspicions in MSBP often involves careful documentation and review of the patient's medical history, including laboratory results, imaging studies, and hospital records. In some cases, covert video surveillance has been used. M. Night Shyamalan's movie "The Sixth Sense" depicts a scene in which Cole (played by Haley Joel Osment) produces a videotaped recording of an adolescent girl deliberately poisoned by her mother. Medical professionals entangled in the web of suspense surrounding MSBP may feel as though they, too, are characters in a powerful supernatural horror movie.

Strong clinical doubt about the validity of a child's symptoms can trigger an investigation by the authorities: law enforcement and child protective services (CPS) agencies. As mandated reporters, hospital personnel are bound by law to report possible child abuse, and they are afforded considerable latitude even if they get it wrong, as long as the report is made in good faith. In light of the horrible crime of child abuse, there must be tolerance for error in reporting it. The difficult question is: How much error is permissible? How much leeway do we give providers before we hold them accountable for inaccurate reporting?

The answer is: it depends, and the margin of error is determined on a case-by-case basis – now that the jury has ruled in the case of Maya Kowalski. Hers is famous for the repercussions of reporting an incorrect diagnosis of MSBP, as featured in the Netflix documentary "Take Care of Maya." The verdict directed compensatory and punitive damages for the Kowalski family due to flawed reporting by medical authorities, and it reminds us of the importance of careful diagnosis, collaborative consultation, attention to all perspectives, attention to consensus, family meetings as informing sessions, and appropriate documentation.

Maya's case made national headlines in 2016 because her doctors were skeptical of her diagnosis of complex regional pain syndrome (CRPS) and, instead, called the state abuse hotline to report Maya's mother, Beata Kowalski, for suspected child abuse. Following a child protection investigation, Maya, then 10 years old, was removed from her family and sheltered at St. Petersburg-based Johns Hopkins All Children's Hospital. Beata died by suicide – she hung herself in the family garage – after being separated from Maya for 87 days.

Accusations of MSBP were never proved, and the Kowalski family sued the hospital in 2018 for false imprisonment, negligent infliction of emotional distress, medical negligence, battery, and other claims. The case took years to reach trial and lasted two months, ending in November 2023. Maya and her father and brother were awarded $261 million in damages. The three broke down crying as the jury read the verdict. (One day later, Maya filed a criminal complaint alleging she was sexually abused during her time at the hospital.)

Maya's case may be settled for now, but the story doesn't end in the courtroom. It leaves us with several uneasy questions. For example, Sally Smith, MD, is a pediatrician and the former medical director of the child protection team who was called to investigate the child abuse allegations against Beata. Smith was vilified in the Netflix movie, and she has been accused of too hastily diagnosing cases of suspected child abuse, "ripping apart families."

It was also alleged in the documentary that Smith was not forthcoming about her role and identity in the investigation, and that she worked for a third party that stood to gain financially from treating medically abused children (Smith and her employer settled with the family in 2022). Should we consider Smith the real Munchausen, inflicting harm upon the entire Kowalski family, and others?

I wonder whether the outcome for the Kowalski family would have been different had the medical team decided that Beata was overzealous about Maya's treatment – for example, demanding ketamine for pain – and that her actions were misguided yet not fabricated and deceptive, as required for a diagnosis of FDIA according to the Diagnostic and Statistical Manual of Mental Disorders, Fifth Edition, Text Revision (DSM-5-TR). The distinction between the unintended medical sequelae of helpful treatments demanded by an overbearing mother and a mother with MSBP who intentionally causes harm in her child is real and has far-reaching implications.

Did the medical team take into account that Beata was a registered nurse and that her advocacy for Maya, which the team interpreted as aggressive, was what any aggrieved mother might do, especially one raised in Poland, where cultural communication tends to be blunt and direct? What about Beata's psychological testing, which showed no evidence of psychopathology other than an "adjustment disorder," as would be expected in someone under duress. If hospital personnel doubted Beata's account that Maya had CRPS, why did they bill for services under that diagnosis?

Also, what about parents' rights to decide the best treatment for their children? This issue is raging not only in the care of very sick children but also children and adolescents diagnosed with gender dysphoria seeking

gender transition therapy. Who decides whether treatment can proceed –
the state, by virtue of increasingly restrictive laws, or the patient and their
family along with the doctor?

What is the correct course of action in cases of MSBP? Remove the child
and traumatize a potentially innocent family, or do nothing and potentially let a child die? Error could lead to false positives (when hospital staff
suspect mental health issues) or false negatives (when staff have difficulty
believing that the mother could be harming her child for unsavory reasons). Those of us in the helping professions (medical, social work, CPS
agencies) must do our absolute best with the tools and resources we have.
Maya Kowalski's case reminds us that there is really no margin for error
in diagnosing medical child abuse. The consequences of a misdiagnosis for
both the child and the family are too steep. It cost Beata Kowalski her life.

34.
Clinical Decision-Making is a Thorn in My Side

"I need a drink and a quick decision. Now it's up to me, ooh, what will be."
– Hall & Oates (from "She's Gone")

As I discussed in the preceding essay, there is inordinate tension deciding between a sick child and one whose symptoms are caused by a family member, however unthinkable that might be. This situation highlights the need for physicians to carefully consider multiple factors in their decision-making process, often making medicine more of an art than a science (see essay 32).

I have faced many thorny clinical situations in my career, and there were times I wished I could have pushed the pause button to have a drink rather than be forced into pushing the panic button and making a quick decision. Here are some additional examples of those "fine lines" that can challenge medical decision-making.

1. Balancing Treatment Quantity and Quality of Life: A common fine line is deciding when to continue aggressive treatment for a serious illness like cancer, versus when to focus on palliative care, ensuring comfort and symptom management, rather than life extension. This balance is often a delicate one, as aggressive treatment may result in side effects that negatively impact a patient's quality of life (QoL).

- In this situation, physicians must communicate effectively with the patient, discussing the potential benefits and drawbacks of each treatment option. The patient's values, preferences, and goals should guide the decision-making process. Balancing treatment and QoL often involves making difficult decisions, but these decisions should always be patient-centered, respecting the patient's autonomy and wishes.

2. **Confidentiality and Safety**: Another example is the fine line between patient confidentiality and the need to share information for the safety of the patient or others. For instance, if a patient is a danger to themselves or others, a doctor may need to breach confidentiality. As a psychiatrist treating potentially dangerous patients, I have found myself in this situation many times.

- The Tarasoff decision was a landmark ruling made by the Supreme Court of California in 1976, in the case of Tarasoff v. Regents of the University of California. The decision held that mental health professionals have a duty to protect individuals who are being threatened with bodily harm by a patient. This may involve warning the intended victim, notifying the police, or taking other necessary steps to protect the potential victim of the harm. The case arose after a patient told his psychologist that he intended to kill Tatiana Tarasoff, but the psychologist did not warn her. Tarasoff was later killed and her parents sued the psychologist and various other employees of the university. The court ruled in favor of the parents, establishing the duty to protect.

3. **Autonomy and Beneficence**: Physicians often walk a fine line in respecting a patient's autonomy (their right to refuse treatment or make deci-

sions about their health) and beneficence (the duty to act in the patient's best interest).

- A doctor may recommend a specific treatment for a patient with a chronic condition, such as diabetes, because they believe it's the most effective way to manage the disease and improve the patient's QoL. However, the patient may want to pursue a course of action that the physician believes is not in their best interest. In such scenarios, it's critical to have open, honest discussions about the risks, benefits, and alternatives, to help the patient make an informed decision that respects their autonomy while also promoting their well-being.

4. **Overdiagnosis and Undertreatment**: There's a fine line between over-diagnosing (and potentially overtreating) patients, which can lead to unnecessary anxiety and medical intervention, and undertreating or missing a diagnosis, which can lead to harm.

- For example, prostate-specific antigen (PSA) testing can lead to overdiagnosis of prostate cancer. Many detected cancers are slow-growing and would not have caused any symptoms or death in the patient's lifetime. However, once diagnosed, patients may undergo treatments like surgery or radiation, which can have significant side effects like impotence and incontinence, as well as pain. Subsequently, patients may not receive adequate pain relief due to concerns about opioid addiction (discussed next), lack of access to multidisciplinary pain management programs, or inadequate assessment and monitoring of pain.

5. **Opioid Prescription**: Physicians must balance the need to manage severe pain with the risk of overprescribing opioids, which can lead to addiction, or avoiding opioids, which can leave patients with unresolved pain.

- A patient recovering from major surgery may initially be prescribed opioids to manage severe postoperative pain. The physician would closely monitor the patient's pain levels and adjust the dosage as needed, with the goal of tapering off the opioids as the pain subsides. The patient would also be educated about the risks of opioid use and the importance of taking the medication exactly as prescribed. If the patient continues to experience pain after the acute postoperative period, the provider might explore non-opioid pain management strategies, such as physical therapy or non-opioid medications. In this way, healthcare providers can help manage severe pain effectively while minimizing the risks associated with opioid use.

6. **End-of-Life Decision Making**: Decisions regarding withholding or withdrawing life-sustaining treatments are often challenging, balancing the prolongation of life against the QoL and the patient's wishes.

- Consider a patient with advanced cancer who has been unresponsive to treatment. The oncologist might suggest a new experimental therapy that could potentially extend the patient's life but comes with severe side effects. The patient, however, values "quality over quantity" and does not wish to endure further discomfort or loss of independence. The experimental treatment is declined. Ultimately, the physician's goal is to ensure that the patient's care aligns with their values and wishes, and that they are able to live their remaining time in the most meaningful and comfortable way possible.

Michael Crichton compared making medical decisions to making movies. He said: "A medical student always is in the position of not knowing how to do something. Medicine also got you into the frame of mind of dealing with very high-pressure situations, dealing with complex factors, emergencies. You often had to act and make fast decisions. Something is always going wrong in a movie, and that kind of experience is invaluable in salvaging a situation."

Navigating thorny medical issues is a great test of our personal resolve because, ironically, it requires instances when we must relinquish control of our power and embrace limits in decision-making, sometimes with great anguish. The sober acknowledgment of our intellectual and clinical finitude as clinicians is one of the most uncomfortable exercises we can undertake in the process of medical decision-making, self-reflection, and becoming a physician.

35.
Corporate Promises Mean Nothing Unless They Have Staying Power

Human resources best practices should include "stay" interviews.

"Stay" is a doo-wop song written by Maurice Williams in 1953 and recorded in 1960 by Williams with his group The Zodiacs. It's simple message – *"Stay, ah, just a little bit longer. Please, please, please, please, please..."* Williams wrote the song when he was only 15 years old. He was attempting to persuade his date to disobey a 10 p.m. curfew.

Commercially successful versions were later also issued by the Hollies, Frankie Valli & The Four Seasons and Jackson Browne. Browne altered the lyrics and sequenced the song to follow "The Load-Out," begging his audience to stay for an encore.

I have worked for many organizations in my career; only two have asked me to "stay." Don't get me wrong. The others didn't fire me – they just never asked me to "stay" – and the first time I was asked to "stay," it backfired. Let me explain.

It was around the turn of the century – the 21st century. I was working for a large midwestern health insurance company. I was a corporate medical director and VP of Behavioral Health, a newly created position designed to better manage care delivery and third-party relationships. I was lured from my roots in Philadelphia, and the company gave me a worthwhile salary and perks, including stock and stock options. I was feeling important. After years of false promises hoping for an executive job, I felt as though my career had finally turned a corner. Maybe one day I would even become the chief medical officer (CMO). That day came and went in a flash.

The company suffered financial losses, and naturally investors were not happy. So, the CMO was fired – actually scapegoated, since financial profitably was not primarily his to manage. The CMO informed each of us – the four corporate VP medical directors – what had happened, and that he was leaving the company. I'll never forget him sobbing on the telephone has he related the events to me. (Today he is a successful medical director and leads initiatives in a multi-state quality improvement organization.)

None of the corporate medical directors were promoted into the CMO role. Instead, the company hired a search firm to find the next CMO. All employees at the rank of VP and higher were asked to assemble in the auditorium for a meeting. The CEO wanted to assure everyone that he would set the organization on a path toward profitability again. His main concern was that his lieutenants would leave the company or be poached by other organizations. The CEO announced he was granting each of us a considerable amount of stock, but the stock would vest only if we stayed three years. If we left the company before then, we would lose the stock. It was a classic ploy used by organizations to retain employees.

I took it in stride – a sign that the company wanted everyone in the auditorium to "stay." It was a form of job security, and given the high turnover of physician executives, I welcomed both the gesture and the payoff for staying on board. About six months later, a new CMO had been found and hired. One of his first orders of business was to lay off all but one of the corporate medical directors. I was not a survivor. The CEO's assurance to retain us, and his offer of goodwill, vanished. It was a false promise.

I harbored considerable resentment toward medical corporations afterwards. I looked out for myself and managed my career as if I were a "company of one." You can imagine my skepticism when a subsequent employer, also a health insurance company, embarked on a "stay" campaign without any apparent motive other than to say: "We truly appreciate you and would like you to stay with the company. What will it take?"

My "stay" interview was conducted by the CMO, a kinder, gentler soul than the midwestern CMO. He asked four questions:

1. What's the most valuable thing about this job that keeps you here?

2. What is the one thing about your job that most makes you think about looking around for another job?

3. What would you like to be doing here or elsewhere over the next 5 to 10 years?

4. What could I (the CMO) do to make your job better?

Stay interviews were conducted throughout the organization. They were meant for listening, not necessarily for immediate problem solving. The goal was not to provide performance feedback; the stay interview was not a performance review. Collective feedback was filtered to the executive leadership team to help make the organization the best possible place to work.

Soon after the interviews were conducted, the three corporate medical directors – me, my CMO, and another medical director – met with the CEO and COO of the company. The CEO and COO were genuinely interested in our concerns and, more importantly, in retaining us. Everyone found common ground and agreed on certain areas in need of improvement that would aid in our retention. An action plan was developed with goals, objectives and a time frame for completion.

This was the first time in my long career that I had the opportunity to participate in a stay meeting. It was a refreshing approach to understanding individual and organizational problems and preventing them from festering and causing individuals to leave the company. While exit interviews can glean essential information, they come too late to retain valuable employees.

A stay interview is preferable because it asks current employees why they continue to work for the organization. The organization does not require a financial or other crisis to proactively engage its workers. By gathering employees' perspectives on the best and worst parts of their jobs, employee morale can be increased, turnover can be reduced, job experience can be improved, relationships with executive leaders can be fortified, and healthcare organizations can find themselves in a much better position to improve employees' lives and strengthen the people and communities they serve.

In order for stay meetings to be successful, organizations must promote trust and open communication and commit to making positive changes. If the organization's climate lacks trust, it needs to rebuild that trust before meaningful stay interviews can be held. Stay interviews would never have worked at my former company because staff turnover was too high, and morale and profitability were too low. Any promises made would be considered empty and unreliable in this type of culture.

While many physicians retire due to age, others have chosen early retirement due to the current state of the U.S. health system. And too many young or midcareer physicians intend to leave their organizations within several years. With the ongoing physician shortage in medicine, finding ways to identify and address doctors' intent to leave a health care organization is vital – and it may require innovative actions by human resources departments. Stay interviews are one such example.

Maurice Williams' original recording of "Stay" remains the shortest single ever to reach the top of the Billboard chart, at 1 minute 36 seconds. By 1990, it had sold more than 8 million copies. It is unfortunate that "stay" has not lived up to its name in the world of human resources best practices. This ideal has not reached a proverbial high note like the song, which, in addition to its soaring sales, employed falsetto for the chorus.

36.
Out of Touch

"Tell me, in a world without pity
Do you think what I'm askin's too much?
I just want something to hold on to
And a little of that human touch..."
—Bruce Springsteen ("Human Touch")

There probably isn't a doctor alive who hasn't heard the term "the laying on of hands." The phrase has its origins in various medical, religious and cultural traditions and has been used to describe a range of practices, including spiritual, ceremonial, and therapeutic gestures.

In contemporary medical contexts, the term is sometimes used more metaphorically to describe the physical examination or hands-on aspects of healthcare. For instance, a physician might use their hands to examine a patient, palpate for abnormalities, or perform certain medical procedures. The term "laying on of hands" has also been used to describe the physical act of touching and the belief in the therapeutic or healing power of touch.

In religious traditions, especially in Christianity, the "laying on of hands" is a ritualistic practice mentioned in the Bible. It is associated with activities such as healing, blessing, and the transmission of spiritual gifts. For example, in the New Testament, there are references to the laying on of hands for healing the sick or bestowing blessings.

Many cultures throughout history have incorporated some form of the laying on of hands in healing rituals. Practices such as Reiki involve the laying on of hands as a method of channeling healing energy. The word "Reiki" is composed of two Japanese words: Rei which means "God's Wisdom or the Higher Power" and Ki which is "life force energy." So, Reiki is actually "spiritually guided life force energy." Practitioners believe that the transfer of energy through touch can promote physical, emotional, and spiritual well-being.

The application of hands can even be seen in medical science fiction. Star Trek's Mr. Spock united with individuals through his hands in a "mind meld" to establish a direct, telepathic link. This allowed the Vulcan to share thoughts, memories, and experiences, or to perceive those of the other person. Spock performed the mind meld by placing his hands on specific points of the subject's face and concentrating to establish the mental link to help that individual in some way. Spock was even capable of melding with a silicon-based creature known as the "Horta" to save it from extinction (season 1, episode 25).

It's important to note that while the "laying on of hands" in a spiritual or metaphysical sense isn't commonly employed in modern medicine, physical touch is still an important, albeit less emphasized, part of healthcare. Touch is mainly used in the physical examination of patients, physiotherapy, wound care, osteopathic manipulation, and other procedures where it is necessary and clinically justified. The practice of medicine has gradually moved away from the "laying on of hands" for several reasons:

1. **Scientific Advancement**: Contemporary medicine is based on scientific evidence and measurable outcomes. While the "laying on of hands" may provide comfort and a sense of healing, there is limited scientific evidence to support the effectiveness of human touch in treating physical ailments.

2. **Professional Boundaries**: Physical touch can be a sensitive issue in healthcare. It's important for healthcare professionals to maintain appropri-

ate boundaries to ensure patient comfort and prevent any potential harm or misinterpretation such as sexual advancements.

3. **Infection Control**: In today's healthcare environment, infection control is a top priority. Unnecessary physical contact can potentially lead to the spread of disease, particularly in a hospital setting.

4. **Cultural Sensitivity**: In our multicultural society, healthcare providers must respect a variety of beliefs and customs. Some patients may not be comfortable with the practice due to personal or cultural reasons.

5. **Alternative Therapies:** While some medical professionals incorporate touch in their practice, there has been a rise in alternative and complementary therapies that specifically focus on touch, such as massage therapy, chiropractic care, and certain forms of energy healing. Patients seeking these therapies may do so outside the traditional medical system.

6. **Technology:** With the advancement of medical science and technology, there has been an increased reliance on diagnostic tests, imaging, and other non-invasive methods. These tools provide valuable objective data, and the emphasis on evidence-based medicine has sometimes shifted the focus away from traditional hands-on examination.

7. **Specialization of Medicine:** As medicine has become more specialized, physicians often focus on specific organ systems or diseases. While hands-on examination remains important, some specialists may rely more on specialized tests and procedures related to their field.

8. **Legal and Ethical Considerations:** Concerns about patient privacy, consent, and avoiding any perception of impropriety have led to more formalized procedures in medical examinations. Healthcare providers are often trained to obtain informed consent and respect patients' boundaries.

Despite these trends and the slate of physician sexual assault cases that have come to light, some patients yearn for good old-fashioned touching, and they feel cheated when their doctor simply does a quick check of their heart and lungs. From the doctors' perspective, many still believe that touch makes important connections with patients.

Simon D. Spivack, MD, MPH, a pulmonologist affiliated with Albert Einstein College of Medicine and Montefiore Health System in New York, remarked, "touch traverses the boundary between healer and patient. It tells patients that they are worthy of human contact .... While the process takes extra time, and we have precious little of it, I firmly believe it's the least we can do as healers – and as fellow human beings."

Spivack concluded: "So in our increasingly technology-driven future, I am quite comfortable predicting that nothing – not bureaucratic exigencies, nor virtual medical visits, nor robots controlled by artificial intelligence – will substitute for this essential human-to-human connection."

Captain Kirk informed Dr. McCoy that the Horta was comprised of stone. When Kirk asked McCoy to heal the Horta, McCoy snapped, "I'm a doctor, not a bricklayer!" McCoy's ingenuity, however, led to a remedy: he applied cement to the creature's wounds. The cure was touch.

37.
Is Creativity the "Sweet Spot" Between Reality and Psychosis?

Reality → Creativity ← Psychosis

We sat (virtually) in our creative writing class talking about – what else – creativity. As you can imagine, there were various perspectives on this topic. From the comfort of my home office, hidden from view below my chest while on a Zoom call, I was doodling on scrap paper and I came up with a symbolic representation of the relationship between reality, creativity and psychosis, as it appears above.

I inserted my primitive drawing in the chat box for my classmates and instructor to see. My instructor asked me to explain it.

"I think creativity can be viewed as a 'sweet spot' between reality and psychosis," I said. "The idea is that creative individuals often think outside the box, breaking from reality in imaginative and innovative ways, which could be perceived as a form of controlled psychosis. It's like taking hallucinogens to achieve a creative state [see essay 16]."

There wasn't much reaction from the class except the emoji of a pair of clapping hands dashing across the visual field.

"Interesting interpretation," my instructor remarked. And that was that. We went on to another topic. But my thoughts reverted to the symbol I had drawn. Can creativity be considered the "sweet spot" between reality and psychosis? I felt as though I needed to explore that possibility further, resorting to the medical literature and relying on my psychiatric experience.

Creativity and psychosis are distinct concepts, and research on this topic cautioned me about making direct connections between them. Creativity generally refers to the ability to generate novel and valuable ideas, while psychosis is a mental health state characterized by a disconnect from reality, often involving hallucinations, delusions, and impaired thinking.

While there is some historical speculation about a link between creativity and mental illness, the relationship is complex and not fully understood. Some famous artists and thinkers have struggled with mental health issues, but it's not accurate to say that creativity is a result of psychosis or that the two exist on a spectrum. Many creative individuals do not have any mental health issues, and many individuals with mental health issues are not necessarily more creative.

I've treated patients in manic episodes. They present with expansive thinking, flight of ideas, pressured speech, and grandiose delusions. They may seem creative – energized and exuberant – but invariably the intensity and duration of their symptoms cause them to appear incoherent or confused. Their thinking, overall, is illogical and disorganized. Their behavior is bizarre and abnormal. They engage in activities that represent a severe departure from reality and are potentially harmful to their reputation. This is the type of behavior psychiatrists label "psychotic."

Creativity, on the other hand, involves thinking outside conventional boundaries, exploring new ideas, and making unusual connections, but these processes are not necessarily indicative of psychosis. Creativity is not a mental disorder. While it's true that some studies have found a correlation between creativity and certain mental health conditions, such as bipolar disorder and schizophrenia, correlation does not imply causation.

Creativity is a multifaceted and complex trait with various contributing factors, including cognitive abilities, personality traits, and environmental influences. Although creativity does involve a parting from conventional ways of thinking, which could be likened to a mild form of psychosis, I don't think it's accurate or helpful to equate the two. The relationship between creativity, reality, and mental health is complex and not fully understood, and it's crucial to avoid oversimplifying or stigmatizing these concepts.

While our Zoom class was proceeding, my attention was diverted else-where as I continued doodling and daydreaming. You could say I was in an altered state somewhere between Reality → Creativity ← Psychosis. Freud would have said that the doodles and daydreams might represent repressed wishes or conflicts, and that these unfulfilled wishes could be traced back to my early childhood experiences. Analyzing them could help reveal underlying psychological issues.

Freud also believed that doodles and daydreams were "windows into the unconscious." In psychoanalytic theory, when repressed unconscious ma-terial surfaces into consciousness, it can cause distress and potentially symptoms that might resemble psychosis. For example, a person might experience intense anxiety, irrational fears, or obsessions. However, these symptoms are not equivalent to the symptoms of genuine psychotic dis-orders like schizophrenia.

Contemporary psychology and neuroscience have offered different perspec-tives on phenomena like doodling and daydreaming. Modern psychology views doodling as a simple, spontaneous act of drawing that can help im-prove concentration, particularly during boring tasks. (Lectures? Boring? LOL!) It's seen as a way to keep the brain engaged rather than an expression of unconscious thoughts or desires. Some research suggests that doodling may help with memory retention and problem-solving.

Contemporary neuroscience has discovered that daydreaming engages a specific network in the brain known as the default mode network (DMN). This network is active when the mind is at rest and not focused on the outside world, such as during daydreaming. Rather than being seen as a form of wish fulfillment, daydreaming is now understood as a state in which the brain consolidates memories and plans for the future. It's considered a crucial aspect of human cognition.

It's interesting, sometimes comical, how the creative process works. I had no idea what I was going to write about in this essay other than I wanted to address the symbol I doodled in class: Reality → Creativity ← Psychosis. Writing without thinking it through beforehand allowed me to be spontaneous. It would not be incorrect to say that spontaneity is often considered a form of creativity. Spontaneity involves acting on impulse, without planning or consideration of the consequences. In a creative context, it allows for the free flow of ideas and actions, which can lead to innovative and unique outcomes.

Spontaneous creativity is often seen in improvisational art forms, such as music, comedy, and dance. What about writing? I was surprised to learn that spontaneous creativity can play a significant role in writing. It often manifests in the form of free writing, brainstorming, or improvisational writing, where the writer allows their thoughts to flow freely onto the page without worrying about grammar, punctuation, or coherence (refer to essay 13).

Spontaneous creativity can be particularly useful during the initial stages of writing, such as when coming up with ideas or overcoming writer's block (essay 11). It can lead to the generation of unique and original ideas, characters, plots, or themes that might not have been conceived through a more structured approach. Additionally, spontaneous creativity can also play a role during the revision process. It can help writers find new ways to express ideas, solve problems with the narrative, or add depth to characters or themes.

However, while spontaneity can contribute to creativity in writing, it's also important to balance it with discipline and structure. After the initial burst of spontaneous creativity, writers often need to refine their ideas, organize their thoughts, and work on their craft to turn their creative impulses into a coherent, polished piece of writing.

Writing this essay certainly took me through the entire realm of:

Reality → Creativity ← Psychosis.

I hope I hit the sweet spot.

38.
I Competed with My Best Friend in Medical School. It was My Worst Nightmare.

They say competition brings out the best in people. At what price?

In theory, entering medical school with a good friend should be a unique and enriching experience. Friends can become study partners, expand each other's networks, and explore the same paths in terms of clinical rotations, research, and eventual career choices. Because medical school is a transformative period, and personal lives may undergo changes, balancing relationships, family commitments, and career development can be challenging, and friends entering medical school together may be better prepared to adapt to these changes in each other's lives. The level of support, collaboration, and understanding between them will play a significant role in shaping their medical school journey and the evolution of their friendship.

I entered medical school with my best friend and it became my worst nightmare.

I'll call him Danny (not his real name). Danny and I had been best friends since third grade. We had a lot in common: sports, music, and girls. He was six months older than me, and he had better luck than I did in all three categories. I was intensely jealous of him, but he never let on. My jealously motivated me to compete scholastically, and I achieved higher grades than Danny in high school.

Danny stayed at home after graduation and attended a "commuter college." I left town for a large university. Our relationship was on hiatus for several years. However, each knew of the other's interest in medical school. We discussed it all the time sitting next to each other in twelfth grade biology class. That's when I first noticed the academic competition between us. However, our distant relationship during college dissipated that competition – so I thought.

Danny and I were accepted at the same medical school. Driving together daily to school renewed our friendship. We quizzed each other every morning on the way to school, and we spoke by phone every night to see which one of us was ahead or behind in assignments. We pushed each other really hard. Discouraging statements were designed to create an impression that one of us was struggling when that clearly was untrue. We aimed to throw each other off guard and pretend we were falling behind in order to gain an advantage over the other person. Our friendship turned into a fierce rivalry, each trying to outdo the other in the basic science courses.

Our relationship was tested toward the end of the first year. Danny called me in a panic. His fiancée had just broken their engagement. He was too upset to concentrate and study for final exams. The dean gave him a week extension. I consoled Danny – it's what any good friend would do – one who understands that experiencing medical school together means they should share common challenges, triumphs, and milestones, and be there to help deal with any setbacks.

I took the final exams as scheduled and told Danny afterwards that they were not difficult – and I truly meant it. The feedback eased his mind, and a week later he took the exams and did great. This shared experience should have strengthened our bond and created lasting memories. It didn't.

As our third year of medical school approached, our relationship had cooled. Danny and I did not take any clinical rotations together, and we barely saw each other until graduation. At the graduation luncheon, we each received academic awards and were elected into the Alpha Omega Alpha (AΩA) honor medical society. The pressure to excel academically, combined with the limited number of top positions in class rankings, created most of the competition between us. Certainly, our competitiveness in high school was kindling for the raging fire.

At the luncheon, Danny told me he was getting married in a couple of weeks. I wasn't even aware he had been dating someone, much less engaged to be married again. I congratulated Danny and told him I was also getting married. To our surprise, we had planned honeymoons in the same city for the same week. After all, we only had one month to marry and honeymoon before starting our residencies. Coincidentally, Danny and I had the same plane reservations. We said hello on the plane and introduced our respective spouses. We said "let's catch up," and we never did.

Although Danny and I did our residencies in the same city at medical centers separated by less than ten miles, we never spoke again. Our friendship was over for good. Competition killed it. Rather than foster growth, camaraderie, solidarity and any number of positive outcomes a shared experience can create, the stress and workload of medical school put an unbearable strain on our friendship. Our relationship could have deepened, as can happen when two good friends support each other through the rigorous demands of medical school, but instead we grew apart and chose to see each other as competitors rather than partners. Our achievements were quite significant, in medical school and beyond, but we paid a steep price for competing against each other.

Competition involves the complex interplay of various psychological factors. I used competition as a way to measure my social and personal worth, based on how I stacked up against others. I was driven to accomplish goals and improve my competency. People like me with high "achievement motivation" often engage in competition to validate their skills and abilities and overcome insecurities. I also became competitive to prove my worth and boost my self-esteem.

I realize I have a tendency to bring out the competitive spirit in people. When I saw this developing in a subsequent relationship, I kidded a colleague, "do not compete with me," or else it will doom our friendship. (That was 15 years ago, and we are still friends.) Recognizing your inner dynamic is pivotal, as it significantly impacts happiness, stress levels, and relationships. Understanding psychological factors helps in managing competition effectively. While competition aided me in some ways, it was ultimately unhealthy and destroyed my friendship with Danny. No relationship will endure competitive pressures that compromise the well-being of the individuals involved.

Looking back through the eyes of an older, more mature person I see many things I would have done differently. My advice to current medical students is to set personal academic goals, but do not try to outperform your peers. Realize that your classmates are not your competitors; they are potential teammates you can learn from. There is no medical student on earth who knows it all. Pair yourself with students who may complement your weaknesses. I can assure you that many of those students will look toward you in the same way as they begin to recognize your strengths.

Any competition that ensues should be healthy and for self-improvement. Leave your "cut-throat" ways at the doorstep (refer to essay 9). By all means, opt for pass/fail rather than letter grades. Pass/fail reduces stress and anxiety and, in turn, creates a less-competitive atmosphere, leading to an increase in collaboration and overall well-being. Pass/fail grading also lays the foundation for self-regulated learning so important to acquiring new skills beyond medical school. You need not worry about USMLE Step 1 and 2 scores and successful residency placement, as studies have shown no significant difference in outcome between letter grades and pass/fail grading.

Finally, I implore you to strike a balance. Competition should motivate you to excel, but it should not compromise the importance of collaboration and mental health – and certainly not pre-existing relationships. The ultimate goal should be to create a learning environment that fosters personal growth, knowledge sharing, and mutual respect between you and your classmates.

The late John Prine penned the song, "In Spite of Ourselves." It is about two imperfect people who are perfect together. He drinks too much beer and tells corny jokes; she swears too much and puts ketchup on her eggs. They not only look past each other's flaws; they find them endearing. It's a relationship that will last in spite of themselves.

Danny and I did not have that type of relationship. If I could tell him one thing today, it would be that I'm sorry for turning our friendship into a competition. I'm sure Danny would say the same thing.

39.
The Role of Music in Fostering Health and Wellness

"A friend knows the song in my heart and sings it to me when my memory fails."
– Donna Roberts

As a music loving physician – I'm sure you've noticed my many references to rock and roll music and musicians in this book – I believe that music is something that can potentially benefit from womb to tomb. Personally, I have noticed that it positively impacts my mood and the way I go about my day.

Research has consistently shown that music can have a profound impact on our mental and physical health. It's not just about listening to your favorite tunes; it's about how these sounds affect our brains, emotions, and every day health in diverse ways.

The effects of music on health can vary greatly depending on the type of music, the individual's personal preferences, and the context in which the music is listened to. I have compiled a short list of the positive effects of music on physical, psychological, and emotional well-being. Here are some key benefits:

♫ Emotional Regulation: Music has a unique way of tapping into our emotions. A melody can uplift our spirits, calm our nerves, or help us process complex feelings. It's a form of expression that transcends words. Physicians may play music in the background when performing procedures and operations to stay on an even keel.

🧠 Cognitive Enhancement: Music can enhance cognitive functioning, focus, and concentration. Music therapy has been used to assist in cognitive rehabilitation. For stroke survivors, Alzheimer's patients, and those with various neurological disorders, music has shown to help improve memory, attention, and even verbal abilities.

Ψ Psychological Health: Music can help reduce stress by lowering cortisol levels, the body's main stress hormone. Music can evoke positive emotions, uplift mood, and foster a more positive outlook on life. Music therapy is often used as a complementary treatment for anxiety and depression, helping to alleviate symptoms.

🤍 Physical Health: Research indicates that listening to music can help lower heart rate and blood pressure, and improve the recovery rate post-exercise. Music therapy can be an effective adjunct to pain management protocols, helping to reduce perceived pain levels. Music can help improve the quality of sleep by serving as a natural sleep aid. Some studies suggest that music can boost the immune system by decreasing stress hormones and increasing growth hormones.

🌐 Cultural Connection: Music is a universal language. It connects us across cultures and experiences, fostering a sense of community and understanding. By listening to or participating in the music of a certain culture, individuals can feel a deeper connection to that culture and its people. This is evident in various cultural events and festivals where music plays a central role.

The physiological mechanisms by which music fosters good physical and emotional health are complex and multifaceted, involving various parts of the brain and body. Although further research is needed to fully understand the mechanisms underlying these benefits, here are some key points:

1. **Activation of Neurotransmitters**: Music can stimulate the release of several neurotransmitters in the brain, such as dopamine and serotonin, which are associated with feelings of pleasure and happiness. This can help to improve mood and reduce symptoms of depression and anxiety.

2. **Autonomic Nervous System Response**: Music can affect the autonomic nervous system, which controls bodily functions like heart rate and digestion. Slow-tempo music can promote relaxation by slowing heart rate and breathing, while fast-tempo music can stimulate these responses.

3. **Stress Hormone Reduction**: By lowering cortisol levels, music can help to reduce feelings of stress and anxiety.

4. **Pain Perception**: Music can affect the brain's limbic system, which is involved in pain perception. This can help distract the brain from pain signals, reducing the perceived intensity of pain.

5. **Emotional and Cognitive Processing**: Music can activate the brain's emotional processing areas, helping individuals to process and express their emotions more effectively. Some types of music can stimulate the brain and enhance cognitive functions like memory and attention.

6. **Social Bonding**: Participating in group music activities can lead to the release of oxytocin, a hormone associated with social bonding and trust.

7. **Immune System Boost**: Some studies suggest that music can enhance the immune system by increasing the production of antibodies and activating immune cells.

I often listen to music in the car to relax during long drives or traffic congestion. I used to listen to the news, but music is more enjoyable and keeps me sane. I'd rather listen to music while driving than do conference calls – any day!

Stephen Klasko, MD, MBA, has been my friend since junior high school. He is passionate about music. In his book, *Feelin' Alright: How the Message in the Music Can Make Healthcare Healthier*, Klasko draws on his experiences as a healthcare executive to demonstrate the emotional power of music as a motivator for building a better healthcare system.

Klasko remarked, "[A]s the president and CEO of Thomas Jefferson University and Jefferson Health [in Philadelphia], my radical communication strategy included a playlist that became a good part of my connection with the 35,000 people who worked for that organization." Among his personal favorite were:

- "Take It to the Limit" by The Eagles

- "Under Pressure" by Queen and David Bowie; and one of my favorites:

- "Human Touch" by Bruce Springsteen (see essays 22 and 36)

When it comes to our health, let's not underestimate the power of a good melody. It's time we embrace music not just as a form of entertainment, but as a companion in our journey towards mental and physical well-being.

40.
Burnout on the U.S.S. Enterprise

There is a reason that writers invented Hollywood endings.

The original Star Trek television series, in my opinion, was the best of the franchise. It lasted only three years (1966-1969), but it has retained a cult following. Among its many television "firsts" were the inter-racial kiss between Captain Kirk and Lieutenant Uhura ("Plato's Stepchildren") and possibly the first depiction of burnout, as seen in the two-part episode "The Menagerie."

Originally intended as the pilot, "The Menagerie" was pushed back to the 11th episode in the first season. It featured Christopher Pike as the captain of the USS Enterprise before James T. Kirk had assumed command. Mr. Spock was Pike's science officer, and Dr. Phil Boyce played the role of the starship's medical officer.

In the episode, Mr. Spock surreptitiously takes command of the Enterprise and sets it on an irreversible course to the forbidden planet Talos IV. Spock faces a court martial and risks the death penalty for his actions. It is not until part 2 that we learn that Spock's motive for returning to Talos IV is to give Pike a semblance of a normal life following a horrible space accident that left Pike disfigured and unable to move or speak (the Talosians are capable of restoring Pike through their power of illusion).

One of the most poignant scenes in this classic adventure, written by Gene Roddenberry, the creator of Star Trek, occurs in part 1. Captain Pike asks to see Dr. Boyce for a second opinion as to whether a distress signal coming from Talos IV is real or fabricated by Spock. Boyce enters Pike's room with a doctor's bag containing liquor, and the following conversation ensues:

PIKE: What the devil are you putting in [that glass], ice?

BOYCE: Who wants a warm martini?

PIKE: What makes you think I need one?

BOYCE: Sometimes a man will tell his bartender things he'll never tell his doctor. What's been on your mind, Chris, the fight on Rigel Seven?

PIKE: Shouldn't it be? My own yeoman and two others dead, seven injured.

BOYCE: Was there anything you personally could have done to prevent it?

PIKE: Oh, I should have smelled trouble when I saw the swords and the armor. Instead of that, I let myself get trapped in that deserted fortress and attacked by one of their warriors.

BOYCE: Chris, you set standards for yourself no one could meet. You treat everyone on board like a human being except yourself, and now you're tired and you...

PIKE: You bet I'm tired. You bet. I'm tired of being responsible for two hundred and three lives. I'm tired of deciding which mission is too risky and which isn't, and who's going on the landing party and who doesn't, and who lives and who dies. Boy, I've had it, Phil.

BOYCE: To the point of finally taking my advice, a rest leave?

PIKE: To the point of considering resigning … There's a whole galaxy of [other] things to choose from.

BOYCE: Not for you. A man either lives life as it happens to him, meets it head-on, and licks it, or he turns his back on it and starts to wither away.

PIKE: Now you're beginning to talk like a doctor, bartender.

BOYCE: Take your choice. We both get the same two kinds of customers. The living and the dying.

"We both get the same two kinds of customers. The living and the dying." What a terrific analogy between doctors and bartenders. How true! It makes a great joke: "How are doctors and bartenders alike…"

This scene is also a great backdrop for understanding burnout. Pike believes he is omnipotent. He sets personal standards that are too high. He blames himself for not achieving them. He begins to imagine there is a better life elsewhere, far away from the Enterprise, where he can participate in activities that once were pleasurable, or at least pursue ones that hold promise – and Pike has a whole galaxy to choose from.

Burnout is defined in the 11th edition of the *International Classification of Diseases* as an "occupational phenomenon" rather than a mental health disorder. The syndrome is conceptualized as resulting from chronic workplace stress that has not been successfully managed. It is characterized by three dimensions:

1. Feelings of energy depletion or exhaustion;

2. Increased mental distance from one's job, or feelings of negativism or cynicism related to one's job; and

3. Reduced professional efficacy.

It is important to note that burnout refers specifically to workplace issues and is not considered a mental health disorder, although seeking professional help is crucial if symptoms of burnout persist or lead to feelings of depression or anxiety.

When Star Trek was being filmed in the 1960s, the concept of "burnout" in the context of psychology did not exist. (The term "burnout" was first coined by the American psychologist Herbert Freudenberger in 1974.) Thus, Dr. Boyce's advice to Captain Pike – to "meet life head on," insinuating he should suck it up and continue doing his job – made sense for the time period (forgetting that Star Trek took place in the 23rd century). Plowing through burnout in the 1960s was the obvious way to go. Now we know better, and there are options to deal with burnout, including exploring different career paths.

Who knows what would have become of the Star Trek series had Captain Pike disregarded Dr. Boyce's advice and resigned his position. After all, it was Captain Pike's tragic accident – an accident he sustained *after* Dr. Boyce convinced him to remain as captain of the Enterprise – that effectively ended Pike's career. It proved to be Kirk's good fortune, however, since Kirk was able to succeed Pike as captain and give us two more glorious seasons of Star Trek.

I guess that's why writers invented Hollywood endings – to leave us uplifted and satisfied, with a focus on optimism and resolution.

41.
Catastrophic Failure of Educational Leadership Can Affect Medical Students

There is no defensible context for hate speech.

U.S. Supreme Court Justice Potter Stewart said he can't define pornography, but he knows it when he sees it. Stewart might just as well have been talking about leadership – reflecting the difficulty in providing a precise definition of leadership but suggesting that individuals can recognize ineffectual leadership when they encounter it.

The abject failure of three university presidents to answer a straightforward question – whether calls for the genocide of Jews violates their policies – shows a lack of moral clarity and competent leadership. When asked repeatedly if calling for genocide of Jewish people violates the University of Pennsylvania's rules or code of conduct, Liz Magill, 57, a legal scholar and former University of Virginia provost, said to Republican Representative Elise M. Stefanik of New York: "It is a context-dependent decision."

"Calling for genocide of Jews … is a context-dependent decision?" Stefanik retorted. "This is an easy question to answer 'yes,' Ms. Magill… Conduct meaning committing the act of genocide? This is unacceptable, Ms. Magill."

Virtually identical "context-dependent" answers were given by the presidents of Harvard and MIT.

Virginia Foxx, the Republican congresswoman from North Carolina who chairs the House Committee on Education and the Workforce, which held the hearing on antisemitism on college campuses on December 5, 2023 issued a statement after Magill resigned under pressure:

"Three chances. President Magill had three chances to set the record straight when asked if calling for the genocide of Jews violated UPenn's code of conduct during our hearing on antisemitism. Instead of giving a resounding yes to the question, she chose to equivocate. What's more shocking is that it took her more than 24 hours to clarify her comments [in a video], and even that clarification failed to include an apology to the Jewish students who do not feel safe on campus. I welcome her departure from UPenn."

Many other lawmakers condemned the presidents' hesitancy to declare the genocide of Jews a violation of school policy, instead giving the lame excuse it depended on the context. The legislators said the testimony of university presidents did nothing to assuage their concerns about antisemitism on campus. Pennsylvania governor Josh Shapiro, who is Jewish, commented, "there's something wrong with the policies of Penn that the board needs to get on, or there's a failure of leadership from the president, or both." Former Philadelphia mayor and Pennsylvania governor Ed Rendell simply said that Magill's testimony was "god awful."

Pfizer CEO Albert Bourla slammed testimonies by all three university presidents for failing to "condemn racist, antisemitic, hate rhetoric," citing the congressional appearance as "one of the most despicable moments in the history of U.S. academia." Bourla's grandparents, aunt and uncle perished at Auschwitz. "I was wondering if their deaths would have provided enough 'context' to these presidents to condemn the Nazis' antisemitic propaganda," he added.

Scott L. Bok, chair of the board of trustees at the University of Pennsylvania, was caught in the crosshairs and also forced to resign his position. Before his departure, Bok gave an accurate account of the situation: "Worn down by months of relentless external attacks, [Magill] was not herself ... Over prepared and over lawyered given the hostile forum and high stakes, she provided a legalistic answer to a moral question, and that was wrong."

It just proves that you can't legislate morality, you can't coach leadership, and there is no substitute for common sense. Three of the brightest educators in the world were tripped up by a simple question and hoisted on their own petard. Magill's successor will no doubt be chosen through a sharper lens, one that views antiracist initiatives as less about having a leg up on DEI and affirmative action and more about taking a firm stand against blatant racism and fascism. The Penn chapter of the American Association of University Professors said: "The next president ... must correct what has become a dangerous myth suggesting that the defense of academic freedom and open expression is in any way contradictory to the fight against antisemitism."

In the fallout, I'm wondering how Penn's next president will affect the moral fiber of Philadelphia's medical community, particularly students at Penn's highly regarded medical school, the nation's first. This remains to be seen, although I do lay out an agenda in the next essay.

Failed leadership in an educational setting – medical or otherwise – can have devastating consequences for students. I witnessed this in the aftermath of AHERF, a catastrophic failure of leadership at an academic medical center. Failed leadership in a medical setting can have several potential implications for medical students:

1. **Lack of Direction**: Failed leadership can result in a lack of clear direction, which may lead to confusion and inefficiency. Medical students may not know what is expected of them, leading to stress and anxiety.

2. **Poor Learning Environment**: Leaders are often responsible for creating a supportive and conducive learning environment. If leadership fails, the learning environment may become hostile, leading to decreased motivation and engagement among medical students.

3. **Poor Quality of Education**: In the absence of effective leadership, the quality of education provided to medical students can suffer. This can result in students lacking essential skills and knowledge needed to succeed in the medical field.

4. **Decreased Morale**: Failed leadership can lead to decreased morale among medical students. This can cause a lack of motivation and engagement, which can negatively impact their academic performance.

5. **Unsafe Conditions**: Poor leaders can create fears about students' safety. This is currently the primary concern for Jewish students across college campuses. Joe Hochberg, a student and vice president of Penn's Jewish Heritage Program, told CNN: "Time and time again, I found that Liz Magill and that those who surrounded her were just dropping the ball, completely ignoring Jewish students' asks for protection because we were scared."

6. **Inadequate Preparation for Future Roles**: Leaders often play a crucial role in preparing students for their future roles as doctors. If leadership fails, students may not be adequately prepared for the challenges they will face in their careers.

7. **Ethical Issues**: Poor leadership can also lead to ethical issues. Medical students may not be taught the importance of ethical behavior in the medical field, which can lead to serious consequences in their future practice.

8. **Miscommunication**: In the absence of strong leadership, communication may suffer, leading to misunderstandings and mistakes that could potentially harm patients.

9. **Risk of Burnout**: The stress and pressure caused by failed leadership can increase the risk of burnout among medical students, which can negatively impact their mental health and career longevity.

10. **Poor Reputation**: Finally, a medical institution with poor leadership can develop a bad reputation, which can deter future students and limit opportunities for collaboration and funding. Indeed, one of the central issues faced by all three university presidents was their degree of financial entanglement with countries openly hostile towards Jews.

It is essential that Penn's next president foster strong, supportive, and ethical leadership in education. They must have aerial vision like Paul Simon to be able to see the Mississippi delta "shining like a national guitar," as well as boots-on-the-ground common sense to know the plain difference between right and wrong.

42.
A Test of Medical Leadership for Penn's New President

The struggles to overcome antisemitism on the campus of the University of Pennsylvania can be used as an example for physicians to harness their untapped potential to become highly visible leaders and change agents.

When the University of Pennsylvania's president Liz Magill was forced to resign her position due to her equivocal stance regarding antisemitic harassment on Penn's campus, J. Larry Jameson, MD, PhD, was soon announced as her interim successor. Jameson had served as executive vice president of Penn's health system and dean of the Perelman School of Medicine since 2011.

Jameson is a prominent molecular endocrinologist, author of over 350 scientific articles and chapters, and an editor of the venerable Harrison's Principles of Internal Medicine. He has garnered a reputation as a strong, thoughtful leader, criticizing U.S. News & World Report's medical school methodology rankings and joining Harvard, Stanford, and Columbia in refusing to participate in the rankings process. (After ending its participation, Penn rose from No. 6 to No. 2 on the 2023-2024 U.S. News Best Medicine School Rankings).

In addition, under Jameson's leadership, Penn's Perelman School of Medicine entered a partnership with historically Black colleges and universities in an effort to attract students from racial groups that are underrepresented in the medical field. Several other initiatives were launched that received recognition for excellence in diversity, equity, and inclusion in medical education and patient care.

Jameson has been lauded by senior faculty and seems to have all the right stuff to assume interim and perhaps permanent leadership at Penn. He has denounced calls for genocide as a form of hate, writing "I want to reiterate that every person at Penn should feel safe and be secure in the knowledge that hate has no home here." But Jameson faces several significant challenges setting a course correction.

The first is to keep Penn academically free from external forces and undue influence by wealthy donors and graduates of Penn's prestigious Wharton School of business. Billionaire Marc Rowan, who co-leads Wharton's board of advisors and donated $50 million to the business school in 2018, is probing Penn's operations, asking questions about their teaching methods, faculty hiring practices, free speech, and political orientation.

Rowan is the deep-pocketed donor who started the successful effort to remove Liz Magill even before the Congressional hearing. After her departure, Rowan submitted a list of 18 questions in an email to Penn's trustees titled "Moving Forward." There is fear among Penn's faculty that Rowan and other philanthropists will attempt to wrest control of Penn's direction and turn it into something other than a university, or at least force the university to be more responsive to pressures from donors. Likewise, there is a congressional movement to hold private schools like Penn accountable for their actions across the board.

One of the questions Rowan is seeking to answer is: "What is the University's policy on direct and indirect foreign donations from countries/ individuals and, specifically, what is the policy on publicly identifying any such contributions? Similarly, what is the University's policy on direct and indirect foreign donations to student organizations?"

This is similar to a question posed to Magill at the Congressional hearing. But whether Penn is deeply financially entangled with countries openly hostile to Jews, or beholden to wealthy Jewish individuals stateside, makes little difference. Jameson will have to disentangle this nebulous web of influence as one of his first orders of business

The second tall order is to immediately restore safety for Jewish students – indeed, for all who feel threatened on campus – and take a firm stand against mounting antisemitism on college campuses. Here is where medical leaders like Jameson can shine, contributing to the reversal of antisemitism not only at his university but also in the medical profession and U.S. medical schools, which has a deplorable history, particularly in the early and mid-20th century.

In the late 19th and early 20th centuries, Jewish immigrants from Eastern Europe began to make significant contributions to the American medical field. However, they faced social and professional discrimination, which was often institutionalized in the form of quotas.

In the 1920s and 1930s, many U.S. medical schools implemented policies to limit the number of Jewish students. These included outright quotas, such as those at Harvard, Cornell, Columbia, and Yale, as well as more covert measures such as "geographic diversity" requirements, which were designed to disadvantage applicants from urban areas with large Jewish populations.

Discrimination also extended to the professional sphere. Jewish doctors were often denied positions in hospitals and medical schools, and professional organizations such as the American Medical Association (AMA) were slow to condemn these practices.

The situation began to improve after World War II, as the horrors of the Holocaust led to a broader societal rejection of antisemitism. In New York State, the Education Practices Act of 1948 set a precedent for other states to pass legislation to eliminate discriminatory admissions practices. Also, in 1948, the Association of American Medical Colleges (AAMC) adopted a policy opposing discrimination on the basis of race, religion, or national origin. However, The AMA and AAMC did little to investigate or condemn the quota system.

As the wave of antisemitism began to lessen and the need for physicians grew, medical schools and graduate medical education programs started to remove the quota systems, and most were eliminated by 1970, according to medical historian Edward C. Halperin, MD, MA, who is also Chancellor and CEO of New York Medical College. In fact, by increasing the percentage of Jewish students from 5% to 50% between 1948 and 1950, Hahnemann Medical College in Philadelphia was able to improve its performance on Pennsylvania's state medical licensure examination and avoid probation.

However, the legacy of these quotas had long-lasting effects on the medical profession and on the Jewish community. Traces of antisemitism persisted in medicine into the late 20th century and beyond. Shocking antisemitism at the University of Toronto's medical school was recently revealed by Jewish-Canadian physician Ayelet Kuper, MD, DPhil. Her account was published in *Canadian Medical Education Journal*. Just imagine how doctors and doctors-in-training holding these vile beliefs treat or intend to treat Jewish patients in their practice.

Although antisemitism in the medical profession is widely condemned, and diversity and inclusion are key priorities for many medical schools and organizations, the history of antisemitism serves as a reminder of the need for vigilance against discrimination in all its forms.

This leads to the third challenge for Penn, which essentially encapsulates the first two concerns: can the new administration self-govern itself and ease tensions over antisemitism? This may be difficult to accomplish given that the abolition of the Jewish quota in U.S. medical school admissions policies was largely driven by forces external to academic medicine: governmental and societal interventions rather than proactive changes within universities themselves.

In comparing the existence of medical school quotas for Jews to the present alleged discrimination against Asian-Americans – that is, viewing Asians as the "new Jews" insofar as both groups have been targeted as "over-represented" at elite institutions – Halperin said, "It is unlikely that the system will reform itself from within. It is far more likely that higher education will circle-the-wagons to defend itself against allegations of bias. If change is to occur, it will need to come from outside the higher education system."

Perhaps a highly-touted physician like Jameson, with demonstrated leadership skills and moral clarity, as opposed to his predecessor – an attorney who tried to legislate morality and whiffed badly when asked to address the evil of genocide – will have much better success quelling campus protest at Penn while assuring the freedom of academic thought and discourse.

43.
How Can Physicians Become World-Class Leaders?

Physicians must sometimes step into the political fray and address global issues apart from medicine.

As discussed in the previous essay, following the December 5, 2023 Congressional hearing into antisemitic harassment at the University of Pennsylvania, J. Larry Jameson, MD, PhD, became interim university president. Jonathan A. Epstein, MD, was soon named interim dean at Penn's Perelman School of Medicine.

Epstein, 62, is a cardiologist and researcher who trained at Harvard and has been at Penn since 1996, most recently serving as the executive vice dean and chief scientific officer of the medical school. In his new role as interim dean, Epstein will oversee 3,000 full-time faculty at Penn and Children's Hospital of Philadelphia, with responsibilities including research, medical education, and the treatment of patients.

The *Philadelphia Inquirer* asked Epstein whether Penn's medical school and health system were impacted by the recent controversy over antisemitism and free speech. His response was:

"The main mission of the school of medicine is focused on caring for patients and finding cures and science. But we are not immune from the controversies that affect the entire campus, the city, and the country. To that extent, it is disruptive and upsetting to see conflict and pain in the world. That affects our students and our faculty and our staff. But as I walk around the hospital and the campus, I don't see disruptions or other activities. I read more about it in the newspaper."

Epstein's response to the grave problem of mounting antisemitism on college campuses seems incredibly naive and parochial. His comments do not appear to have the substance one would expect from a world-class leader charged with solving hate speech on college campuses and determining what role, if any, should donors play in deciding school policy. Epstein may turn out to be an excellent dean, but if it is true that all physicians are leaders, then someone in his position must inspire others, engage them in action, and have a blueprint and buy-in for change on and off campus.

I believe the problem with many physicians is that they do not view themselves as leaders. They may think, for example, that because the questions raised at the Congressional hearing ultimately reverberate beyond academia, the problem of antisemitism is not their responsibility. But physicians are often looked upon as leaders, and they must have answers to wide-ranging issues far afield from medicine. Shying away from them only perpetuates the myth that physicians cannot lead on the global stage. This begs the question: What skills are required for physicians to leverage their training and experience to become world leaders outside the field of medicine?

1. **Transferable Skills**: Medical leaders possess skills such as decision-making, problem-solving, team leadership, and communication which are transferable to other sectors. These skills can be used to lead teams, organizations, or even countries.

2. **Public Health Policy**: With their in-depth knowledge of public health, physicians can effectively contribute to the development of public health

policies. They can work with governments or international organizations to improve healthcare systems globally.

3. **Education and Research**: Doctors can contribute to the field of education as professors, researchers, or administrators. They can use their expertise to train the next generation of leaders or to conduct research that influences policy and practice.

4. **Philanthropy**: Many medical leaders are involved in philanthropy, contributing their wealth and influence to causes they care about. This can lead to leadership roles in non-profit organizations or foundations.

5. **Health Advocacy**: Physicians can become advocates for health, working to raise awareness about health issues and to influence policy. This can lead to leadership roles in advocacy organizations or in government.

6. **Entrepreneurship**: Doctors can also become entrepreneurs, using their knowledge of the healthcare sector to start their own businesses. This can lead to leadership roles in the business world.

7. **Consulting**: With their knowledge and experience, medical leaders can become consultants, advising governments, organizations, or businesses on health-related issues. This can lead to leadership roles in the consulting sector.

8. **Politics**: Medical leaders can enter politics, using their knowledge and experience to influence policy and legislation. This can lead to leadership roles at the local, national, or international level. There are 19 physicians in the 118th Congress (2023 – present), of whom 15 serve in the House and 4 serve in the Senate.

9. **Global Health Perspective**: Physician leaders often engage in global health initiatives beyond clinical practice. This could involve participating

in international health organizations, contributing to global health policy, or leading initiatives that address health disparities on a global scale.

This list is not all-inclusive. There are many other skills, knowledge, and leadership qualities physicians can leverage to become influential world leaders outside the field of medicine. What's most important is staying informed about global issues, developing a broad perspective, and actively seeking opportunities to contribute to positive change beyond the boundaries of healthcare.

Physicians have transitioned from successful medical careers to become world-class leaders in many fields. Dr. Gro Harlem Brundtland is the former Prime Minister of Norway. She served as the Director-General of WHO from 1998 to 2003. Dr. Brundtland played a key role in climate control and sustainable development. She chaired the Brundtland Commission, which introduced the concept of sustainable development in the report "Our Common Future."

Dr. Paul Farmer (deceased 2022) co-founded Partners In Health, an organization that provides healthcare to impoverished communities worldwide. He was a leader in global health and social justice, advocating for equitable access to healthcare.

Dr. Jim Yong Kim was the 12th president of the World Bank Group from 2012 to 2019. He co-founded Partners In Health with Dr. Paul Farmer and served as the president of Dartmouth College from 2009 to 2012.

Dr. Bernard Lown (deceased 2021) was a renowned cardiologist and inventor of the direct current defibrillator, Dr. Lown co-founded the International Physicians for the Prevention of Nuclear War (IPPNW), which was awarded the Nobel Peace Prize in 1985. His advocacy work focused on nuclear disarmament and peace.

Dr. Ernesto "Che" Guevera (deceased 1967) has the dubious distinction of having his occupation listed in Wikipedia as "guerilla" as well as physician, diplomat, and author. Guevera is best remembered for his role in Cuba's revolution, where he was both revered and reviled. *Time* named Guevera one of the 100 most influential people of the 20th century.

These are just a few examples of physicians who have demonstrated that doctors can leverage their medical expertise and leadership skills to address broader global issues, ranging from public health and sustainable development to diplomacy, peace, and activism. Medical training shaped their leadership views through a lens of compassion for the poor, an understanding of the social determinant of health, and a desire to alleviate disease and suffering. Their diverse contributions showcase the potential for physicians to become influential leaders on the world stage.

44.
Down with Diversity?

For years, scholars have called on institutions of higher learning to recommit themselves to open inquiry and tolerance for diverse viewpoints. What's changed?

I was shocked to learn how universities, large and small, public and private, have been hijacked by extreme right-wing leaders connected directly or indirectly to the GOP. Examples include:

- Youngstown State University bypassed the normal search process to select its new president, Republican U.S. Representative Bill Johnson. Johnson has no experience in academia and voted with dozens of other GOP lawmakers in their failed effort to block Joe Biden's 2020 victory.

- Kevin Guskiewicz left his position as chancellor of the University of North Carolina (UNC)-Chapel Hill partly due to political interference from the university's almost-all-Republican trustees. Guskiewicz was replaced on an interim basis by board trustee Lee Roberts, a former state budget director under a Republican governor. Roberts has a background in finance and real estate, but he has no substantive experience running a large university.

- Meanwhile, in a messy and contentious process, UNC-Chapel Hill initially denied and subsequently granted tenure to Nikole Hannah-Jones, one of America's top Black journalists and a Pulitzer Prize winner for the 1619 Project. Hannah-Jones instead joined the faculty of Howard University.

- Florida's Republican governor and former presidential candidate Ron DeSantis elected Ben Sasse, a Republican senator from Nebraska, president of the flagship University of Florida despite protests related to both the search and Sasse, himself.

- In addition, DeSantis aims to crush the progressive New College of Florida by appointing Richard Corcoran interim president. Corcoran is the former Republican Speaker of the House in Florida's legislature. The decision to hire him occurred before public comments – virtually all negative – were considered.

This academic whitewashing and suppression of educational freedom across America is lamentable. Until right-wing extremism is dismantled and people with a demonstrated history of commitment to liberalism and open discourse are put back in place, the ugly intolerance of diversity we now see on our nation's campuses will reign supreme.

Florida is a prime example of a state where a swath of new conservative trustees has been appointed to colleges through political back-channels, arguing that liberal leanings have corrupted the state's culture. Columnist Will Bunch remarked, "Controlling [university] campuses – curbing their diversity initiatives and downsizing the liberal arts that promote critical thinking while pumping up pro-capitalism business or STEM courses – helps their real agenda, which is molding young people less likely to challenge their authority. We lose that war when they capture Youngstown State…"

Bunch attributes the Republican blowback to a decades-long emphasis on liberal arts education, beginning after World War II with the GI Bill and piquing in the early 1970s with college protests against the Vietnam War. Ronald Regan subsequently marshalled a conservative educational agenda, first in California when he was Governor, and later as President of the United States, making sure that conservative governors and state legislatures slowed taxpayer aid for universities and boosted tuition – a trend that accelerated dramatically after the Great Recession.

Gradually, over the last decade, liberal university trustees have been ousted in the name of "political correctness" or "wokeness." Their conservative replacements have thrown their weight around campus and buddied-up with influential donors bent on steering universities away from liberal ideas and professors, as UNC did in the case of Hannah-Jones.

For example, University of Pennsylvania alumnus Saul B. Rosenthal, who donated approximately $168,000 in scholarships earmarked for financially burdened business students, sued Penn alleging that the school instead gave some of those scholarships to aid student athletes. Well-known billionaire Marc Rowan, who leads Penn's Wharton business school's advisory board, has made no secret about his attempts to alter the school's mission and academic and governance practices, contributing to the recent resignations of Penn president Liz Magill and board chair Scott Bok.

Just when institutions of higher learning seemed to be making strides in the area of diversity, equity, and inclusion (DEI), no sooner were they called to fight for a new kind of diversity: diversity of thought. When the Harvard Institute of Politics removed alum Representative Elise Stefanik (R-N.Y.) from its Senior Advisory Committee in the wake of the January 6 insurrection and her ongoing claims of voter fraud in the 2020 presidential election, Stefanik wrote in a statement: "The decision by Harvard's administration to cower and cave to the woke Left will continue to erode diversity of thought."

Granted the extreme left can at times resemble the extreme right in its adherence to ideological dogma. But I really think Stefanik has it backwards. What's more noticeable in America is the increasingly radical nature of the right-wing anti-intellectual agenda. And a right-wing war against freedom of thought in America is only heating up – it could get a lot worse – and it could further erode freedom of thought and expression in medicine.

I say "further" because we have already witnessed a strong backlash against DEI initiatives in medical schools as well as practice in the form of wresting medical decision-making away from doctors and patients – for example, decisions related to abortion and gender identity and even medical licensure (physicians who comprise states' medical licensing boards are typically political appointees of governors).

There has also been a huge uptick in the number of scholars and physicians who have been sanctioned, or have had attempted sanction, since 2000. Views surrounding COVID-19 policies and vaccination contributed to most of the actions. Sanction attempts were also in response to teaching practices, scientific inquiry, speech about race, and institutional policies.

Mayo Clinic fired internal medicine physician Steven Weiss after he published a book about his experiences treating patients through the darkest days of the COVID-19 pandemic. In fact, physicians' rights to free expression have become so encumbered that it has become necessary to propose a model to distinguish between citizen speech, physician speech, and clinical speech in order to regulate it.

Organizations such as Do No Harm, which ostensibly advocate for patients, continue to file federal civil rights complaints attacking diversity efforts at medical schools and institutions. Their report entitled "The Return of Segregation," attempts to debunk well-established research showing that matching physician ethnicity and patient demographics leads to better healthcare outcomes. But the report simply criticizes published studies as opposed to contributing new empirical evidence about outcomes after patients see physicians of the same race.

The report might have had some merit if it were actually true that racial concordance is unimportant and that matching patients and doctors creates a de facto "segregation" of the races. In the same vein, the HBO documentary "South to Black Power," featuring the *New York Times* opinion columnist Charles M. Blow, calls for Black Americans to move to the South to gain political footholds. I may disagree with Blow, but I do find it enlightening that sparking the conversation about "reverse segregation" could change the power structure in this country.

And that is what must be preserved: the ability to have the conversation.

45.
Is it Noble or Selfish to Never Practice Medicine After Getting a Medical Degree?

Opinions are divided, but it's clear that non-traditional careers are an alternative to practicing medicine.

A Harvard medical school student realized in his third year that he had lost his desire to become a doctor. Nevertheless, the student decided to complete his fourth year and obtain his MD degree. The student is now planning for a career in pharma or even comedy. Some individuals who read his online essay found the student's decision-making comical in itself. Overall, their comments were evenly divided about the student's virtues and next moves.

Before exploring readers' reactions, we ought to know something about this student's reasons for opting out of the medical profession. The student wrote: "Reflecting on the elements that brought me down, I felt sadness for my patients' health, particularly when it seemed their condition could not be cured or treated effectively; disappointment over the influence of insurance coverage in determining which treatments patients received; frustration at the amount of documentation, which seemed to take precedence over time spent with patients; and discouraged by the overall environment where it seemed hospital personnel did not feel valued or happy to be there."

Let's not dwell on the merits of the student's reasons but dive right into readers' reactions to it, whether they shamed or commended him on his decision. I divided the comments into "selfish" and "noble." Here is a sample:

Selfish

- How did this individual get into medical school not knowing his passions? Why did he apply when still intellectually and emotionally immature?

- As someone involved in teaching students and residents throughout my career, I know that an incredible amount of time and resources are devoted to educating doctors, and I find it very distressing when someone uses those resources and never provides care, especially when the provider shortage is so bad.

- Some other student could have really made something of the spot at Harvard medical, but now society is deprived of those benefits. This seems like a very narcissistic thing to do.

- You can be humorous with a bachelor's degree.

- It is somewhat revealing that the [student] states he went into medicine to help others, and yet all the career choices he now describes are designed to help him.

- Now there's comedy. Joining up with the pharmaceutical industry that puts sales above well-being. Trying to advertise the latest and greatest (and most expensive) alternatives to disease management and shying away from promoting healthy behaviors.

- You didn't have the right stuff.

Noble

- With the pharmaceutical path, you may be able to help count-less more people than you could have with the conventional MD route.

- Sounds like the smartest man in the room to me: Do what makes you happy! And avoid the EMR cash register and ham-ster wheel.

- If working with patients and practicing medicine is still a pas-sion, consider using your skills and knowledge at a free clinic; if comedy is your passion, instead, enjoy yourself!

- Follow your heart, and the mind will be of great service to others.

- Everything he says is true. We went into medicine to help people and make the world a better place. But it seems that everything is more important than the patient.

- Good luck! It just proves that there is no other type of study/ education that opens so many possibilities as medicine. Good for you!

- I hope he's finding fulfillment outside the traditional med school to residency pathway, and I'm happy that he's thought-fully making the best choices for him.

The comments do not provide a consensus on whether it is selfish or noble to never practice medicine after medical school. One commentator – not the only one – was able to see the argument philosophically from both sides, writing, "Let's not shame people into staying where they deeply do not wish to be or condemn them based on good faith decisions made when they didn't fully understand what they were getting into."

I think this reader made many good points, so I decided to quote him entirely: "The practical realities of clinical practice as a physician must be experienced to fully appreciate [them]. Pursuing and, if ultimately admitted, getting through medical school is something of a leap of faith for many. Sometimes it turns out to be a bad fit, a realization that may dawn after committing to a lot of debt. Of course, it rankles some given that accepting admission indirectly crowds someone else out (of this scarce resource) and doesn't provide the expected societal return on investment of a practicing clinician. On the other hand, do any of us want a physician who chronically doesn't want to be in that role? He may yet apply his education and degree profitably outside of clinical practice."

Many years ago, I conducted a small study showing that over 90% of students who matriculated in two U.S. medical schools (Temple University and the University of Pennsylvania) graduated in four years. This percentage is in line with the Association of American Medical Colleges, which found that 4-year graduation rates ranged from 81.7% to 84.1%. Still, after six years, the average graduation rate was 96.0%.

Reasons for dropping out of medical school can be diverse, but common ones include academic struggles, financial pressures, personal health or family issues, lack of interest, or, in this instance, a desire to pursue a different career path. It is important to note that the majority of dropout causes are non-academic.

After leaving medical school, former students may pursue a range of alternate career paths. Some may choose to continue their education in a related field, such as public health, biomedical sciences, or health care administration. Others may decide to enter the workforce directly, taking jobs in health care, education, or research. Some will pursue careers distant from medicine or unrelated to it.

Perhaps this student will follow in the footsteps of the Monty Python actor Graham Chapman (1941-1989), who turned down a career as a doctor to be a writer and comedian. I wish this student well, and I do not begrudge him for almost forcing me to go to Mexico for medical school. Well, I never would have had a shot at Harvard anyway.

46.
Is the Medical Profession on Life Support?

Physicians weigh in on the prognosis.

I try to be upbeat about the future of medicine. Admittedly, I've been critical at times, but I've also portrayed medical education and practice in a positive light. Essays 19 through 21, for example, discuss a bright future for medical students, with the only reservation being the extent of their engagement in clinical roles versus nonclinical roles.

I was highly dismayed by the negative reactions I received to these essays when they initially appeared online. To be fair, I decided to summarize the many concerns voiced by the commentators, mostly physicians, including their thinly veiled hostility toward the medical profession. Taken together, their comments make me question whether the field of medicine requires resuscitative measures.

Here, in no particular order, is a sample of what some physicians believe is wrong with the medical profession:

- Absurdly long working hours

- The cynical rule of hospital administrators

222

- Patients' misbegotten beliefs in the "idiocies of alternative medicine"

- Broadly deteriorating working conditions

- Income stolen by fiat

- Revenues that no longer cover the costs of operating a practice

- Insurers who decide how medicine should be practiced

- Patients' beliefs that they are entitled to everything

- Drug manufacturers pricing medications beyond patients' reach

- Tedious medical coding requirements

- Slavery to computers and electronic medical records

- Prior authorization and other administrative hassles

- Faceless bureaucrats making clinical decisions without penalty of law

- Insufficient economic rewards and professional flexibility

- Incessant staring into computer screens at the expense of patient interaction

- Academic medical centers shunning PCPs, regarding them as "medical low life"

- Draconian policies that have taken the fun out of practicing

Here are quotes from two physicians who view retirement as the only solution:

> "It's simply no longer worthwhile to practice medicine; the gratitude and appreciation of my patients can't make up for the depredation of clinical medicine by the government and insurers. I'm glad to look forward to retirement in a few years. I fully expected to practice another decade, but no longer."

> "We certainly live in Bizarro World. Yes, I too am looking forward to retirement this summer after 40 years on the hamster wheel."

Here, in no particular order, is a sample of what some physicians believe is wrong with medical education and up-and-coming doctors:

- They will be less knowledgeable in anatomy and physiology and far less competent in performing physical examinations

- They will be unable to read their own patients' x-rays and MRI studies

- They will be unable to comprehend a scholarly paper or critique it thoughtfully

- They will be shielded from private practice role models

- They will need artificial intelligence to tell them what tests to perform and what the results mean

- They will not read papers and journals in the evenings because such dedication upsets their work-life balance

- They will be business-savvy cogs in a system still dictated by payers and administrators

- They will most likely join a medical group, abdicating personal control of their finances

- They will be culturally competent and committed to everything, but they will be intellectually circumscribed

- They will not recognize when symptoms just don't fit a clinical picture because they are obsessed with empathetic care and patient rankings; but

- They will be warmer, fuzzier, and better at working in groups

Here are a few direct quotes:

> "They'll be politically and culturally homogeneous, lacking any capacity for critical thought, independent query, and will be subject to the political whims of the degree granting institutions they apply to. Or, they'll just be good at lying to get into medical school because they don't actually believe the political litmus test inherent in the personality and behavioral assessments required for admission. Either way, you end up [with] pathological liars, or groupthink that kills scientific innovation and leads to the exact type of stagnation that ensued after Semmelweis was ostracized."

> "Every time the patient will mention a complaint, they will say, with practiced compassion in their voice: 'Oh I'm so sorry to hear that you have X,' then document it in the electronic medical record without actually examining the patient. Then they will report the supervising attending

for telling them: 'Instead of keep saying how sorry you are, why don't you ask more questions…'"

"…a new generation of physicians who are so narcissistic and sensitive to no end caring more about taking selfies, pronouns, woke culture and safe places than taking on the precious role as healer. This is all part of the slow-motion destruction of our healthcare system and its ability to care for patients."

Read my summation in the Afterword.

AFTERWORD

47.
The Fifth Vital Sign

"If you don't take a temperature, you can't find a fever."
—Samuel Shem, The House of God

I enrolled in a creative writing course at a local university to better understand the parameters of narrative medicine. I learned about the pillars of the narrative, such as poetry and creative nonfiction, and our class talked extensively about the healing power of storytelling. Toward the end of the semester, I commented that narrative medicine should be the fifth vital sign, because just like the four traditional vital signs (temperature, pulse, respiration rate, and blood pressure) provide critical information about a patient's physical health, narrative medicine provides direct insight into a patient's emotional, psychological, and social health. It helps the clinician glimpse the patient's personal experience with their illness, fears, concerns, and hopes.

Narrative medicine adds a dimension of care that complements and enriches the information obtained from the traditional vital signs. Just as vital signs can indicate a physical condition that needs immediate attention, narrative medicine can help identify important emotional issues early on. The concept of narrative medicine as the "fifth" vital sign suggests that patients' stories are equally crucial as their physicality for a comprehensive understanding of their health. Why shouldn't personal narratives be considered the fifth vital sign?

Everyone in my class seemed to agree. They liked *The Fifth Vital Sign* as a title for a book about narrative medicine – this book! (The obvious first choice was simply *Narrative Medicine*.) My instructor commented: "The 'fifth' is magic for the alchemists. Mercury is the fifth element [in numerology] and the only one that embodies masculine and feminine (solid and liquid) properties at room temperature. And the fifth anything turns a square into a circle. Quintessential stuff, Art!"

I was puzzled by my instructor's use of the phrase "the fifth anything turns a square into a circle." I had to do some research to decipher its meaning. Metaphorically, in a medical context, if we consider the four corners of a square as the four traditional vital signs, these provide a structured, quantitative assessment of a patient's physical state. Adding a fifth element, such as narrative medicine, introduces a qualitative, humanistic aspect to patient assessment. This "rounds out" the picture, making it more holistic and complete, just as adding a dimension to a square can transform it into a circle (or more accurately, a sphere in a three-dimensional context).

Even my instructor's use of the word "quintessential" was apropos. Ancient Greek philosophers claimed there were five elements: earth, water, air, fire, and a fifth substance that made up objects in the heavens. This idea was passed down through the ages to Latin-speaking scholars who called the fifth element quintessence – from the Latin words quintus, meaning "fifth," and essentia, meaning "being." In the Middle Ages, people believed the *quinta essentia* was integral to all kinds of matter, and if they could somehow isolate it, it would cure all disease. Eventually, the word's meaning evolved into our modern definition: the essence of a thing in its purest and most concentrated form. In other words, the narrative in medicine.

Narrative medicine represents purity because it focuses on the humanistic aspects of medical practice – the personal stories, emotions, social context, and experiences of patients and healthcare providers. It symbolizes the core of medicine, which is not only about diagnosing and treating diseases but also about understanding and empathizing with patients as whole individuals. Narrative medicine embodies the ideal of quintessence – the fifth essence – the most essential part of something. It *should* be considered the fifth vital sign, a useful tool for detecting or monitoring a range of medical problems.

The vitriolic comments in the previous essay bear witness to the problems yet to be solved in the medical profession. It's clear that we are facing ongoing challenges such as burnout, high stress, long hours, increasing healthcare costs, and evolving healthcare delivery models. However, it's essential to note that the state of any profession, including medicine, can be influenced by various factors such as technological advancements, societal changes, economic conditions, and healthcare policies.

The healthcare industry is continually adapting and innovating to meet these challenges. Investments in telemedicine, mental health resources for healthcare workers, and the recognition of the importance of work-life balance are all efforts to support the profession. Yet, while multiple stakeholders are busy addressing these problems, the utility of the medical narrative is virtually overlooked as a viable means to support clinicians and patients through turbulent times. Narrative medicine attests to the healing power of putting words to experience, and it has done so since antiquity by promoting empathy, enhancing communication, fostering reflection, facilitating interprofessional collaboration, informing clinical practice, and educating students.

The third law in Samuel Shem's *House of God* is, "At a cardiac arrest, the first procedure is to take your own pulse." It's a reminder that we need to take care of our own mental and emotional health in order to effectively take care of our patients. We can't rely exclusively on other people to fix medicine's problems. We also need to look inward for a solution by becoming our own patients, scheduling our own personal checkups in which we constantly re-examine ourselves and assess our well-being. Quite simply, we need to monitor our vital signs and place greater emphasis on the fifth vital sign. Narrative medicine is as much a tool for us as it is our patients.

Notes

Preface

1. Chris Adrian "Grand Rounds": https://granta.com/grand-rounds

2. The four genres of narrative medicine: https://www.ncbi.nlm.nih.gov/pmc/articles/PMC3034473

3. Patricia Hampl quote: https://core1section11.files.wordpress.com/2013/02/hampl-memory-imagination.pdf

Essay 1: https://www.kevinmd.com/2023/10/kick-start-your-writing-with-a-surprise.html

Essay 2

1. William Carlos Williams quote: https://www.goodreads.com/author/quotes/15435.William_Carlos_Williams?page=3

Essay 3

1. "The Value and Benefit of Narrative Medicine for Psychiatric Practice": https://www.cambridge.org/core/journals/bjpsych-bulletin/article/value-and-benefit-of-narrative-medicine-for-psychiatric-practice/C8CF7372FF903CD83B55D87D6B738131

2. Carl Jung quote: https://www.goodreads.com/quotes/23089-the-meeting-of-two-personalities-is-like-the-contact-of

3. Michael Crichton quote: https://www.michaelcrichton.com/biography/doctor/

Essay 4

1. Rita Charon on "close reading": https://journals.lww.com/academicmedicine/fulltext/2016/03000/close_reading_and_creative_writing_in_clinical.26.aspx

2. Josephine Ensign quote and reading drill: https://josephineensign.com/2014/07/30/a-narrative-medicine-closer-close-reading-drill

Essay 6: https://www.kevinmd.com/2023/11/lets-close-the-gap-between-physician-writers-and-writers-who-are-physicians.html

Essay 7

1. Rita Charon quote: https://pubmed.ncbi.nlm.nih.gov/11597295

2. Carolyn Roy-Bornstein quote: https://www.medpagetoday.com/opinion/second-opinions/107208?trw=no

3. CDC initiative: https://www.cdc.gov/niosh/impactwellbeing/default.html

Essay 8

1. Denny Zeitlin quote: https://www.denniszeitlinmd.com/a-personal-note.html

2. "Good Clinical Practice": https://www.fda.gov/about-fda/center-drug-evaluation-and-research-cder/good-clinical-practice

Essay 9

1. Survey: https://www.elsevier.com/promotions/clinician-of-the-future-education-edition?utm_source=banner&utm_medium=dg&utm_campaign=cotf&utm_content=srpt#1ackowms1mu2erhf3vhv7u

Essay 11

1. Bob Dylan "Watching the River Flow": https://archive.org/details/simpletwistoffat00gill/page/30/mode/2up

2. Edmund Bergler "Does Writer's Block Exist?": https://www.jstor.org/stable/26301237?seq=1#page_scan_tab_contents

3. Norman Mailer quote: http://www.notable-quotes.com/m/mailer_norman.html

4. Patricia Huston "Resolving Writer's Block: https://www.ncbi.nlm.nih.gov/pmc/articles/PMC2277565/pdf/canfamphys00047-0094.pdf

5. Hugh MacLeod quote: https://sive.rs/book/IgnoreEverybody

6. The Guardian: https://www.theguardian.com/music/2020/jun/20/bob-dylan-rough-and-rowdy-ways-review-enthralling-mischievous-and-very-male

7. Pitchfork: https://pitchfork.com/reviews/albums/bob-dylan-rough-and-rowdy-ways

8. Rolling Stone: https://www.rollingstone.com/music/music-album-reviews/bob-dylan-rough-rowdy-ways-1015086

Essay 12

1. Bill Maher's "Club Random" podcast: https://www.youtube.com/watch?v=k_VtqkQ5MTw

Essay 13: https://www.kevinmd.com/2023/11/bad-grammar-makes-me-mad-i-cant-help-it.html

Essay 14: Adapted with permission from *The Journal of Medical Practice Management*, Volume 29, Number 3, pages 152-156. American Association for Physician Leadership®, 800-562-8088, www.physician-leaders.org

Essay 15: Adapted with permission from *The Physician Leadership Journal*, Volume 9, Number 4, pages 60-65, https://doi.org/10.55834/plj.6245868299. American Association for Physician Leadership®, 800-562-8088, www.physicianleaders.org

Essay 16: https://www.kevinmd.com/2023/11/the-real-story-behind-woodstock-is-not-the-brown-acid.html

Essay 17

1. Jimmy Santiago Baca quote: https://quotefancy.com/quote/1522922/Jimmy-Santiago-Baca-Being-a-human-being-without-forgiveness-is-like-being-a-guitarist

2. James Thurber quote: https://www.amerlit.com/quotations/QUO-TATIONS%20Thurber.pdf

3. David Fear quote: https://www.nytimes.com/2013/12/15/magazine/confessions-of-a-daydreamer.html

4. James Thurber's diagnosis of sympathetic opthalmia: https://jamanetwork.com/journals/jamaophthalmology/fullarticle/270682

Essay 18: https://www.kevinmd.com/2023/10/reflections-on-human-suffering.html

Essay 19: https://www.kevinmd.com/2023/08/the-medical-establishments-fight-for-and-against-diversity.html

Essay 20: https://www.medpagetoday.com/opinion/second-opinions/107258?trw=no

Essay 21: https://www.kevinmd.com/2023/11/the-physician-of-the-future-may-not-be-a-clinician.html

Essay 22

1. ChatGPT answers drug questions: https://www.cnbc.com/2023/12/05/free-chatgpt-may-incorrectly-answer-drug-questions-study-says.html

2. ChatGPT answers epilepsy questions: https://www.seizure-journal.com/article/S1059-1311(23)00300-X/fulltext

3. ChatGPT inaccuracies and quote by researchers: https://jamanetwork.com/journals/jamanetworkopen/fullarticle/2809975

4. AI error rate: https://arstechnica.com/health/2023/11/ai-with-90-error-rate-forces-elderly-out-of-rehab-nursing-homes-suit-claims/?comments=1&comments-page=1

5. Medical educator Bernard S. Chang quote: https://jamanetwork.com/journals/jama/fullarticle/2809659

Essay 23: https://www.kevinmd.com/2023/11/medicine-has-become-the-new-mcdonalds-of-health-care.html

Essay 24

1. Neil Young quote: https://www.yahoo.com/entertainment/neil-young-says-won-t-164418299.html?fr=yhssrp_catchall&guccounter=1

Essay 25

1. Liz Cneyney quote: https://twitter.com/ABC/status/1535055581035241491?ref_src=twsrc%5Etfw%7Ctwcamp%5Etweetembed%7Ctwterm%5E1535055581035241491%7Ctwgr%5E699b5a54c2df1872c1ada1da0897718f64810f0b%7Ctwcon%5Es1_&ref_url=https%3A%2F%2Fabcnews.go.com%2FPolitics%2Fliz-cheneys-mission-donald-trump-white-house%2Fstory%3Fid%3D95379999

2. Capitol riot statistics: https://www.justice.gov/usao-dc/30-months-jan-6-attack-capitol

Essay 26

1. Bruce Springsteen quote: https://www.app.com/story/entertainment/music/2023/02/02/bruce-springsteen-e-street-band-tampa-tour-2023-setlist-review/69844770007

2. Rainbow Bridge: https://www.rainbowsbridge.com/Poem.htm

Essay 28: https://www.kevinmd.com/2023/11/sending-in-tougher-canaries-wont-fix-the-problem-of-physician-well-being.html

Essay 29: Adapted with permission from *The Journal of Medical Practice Management*, Volume 35, Number 6, pages 304-307, American Association for Physician Leadership®, 800-562-8088, www.physician-leaders.org

Essay 30: Adapted with permission from *The Journal of Medical Practice Management*, Volume 39, Number 3, pages 38-43. American Association for Physician Leadership®, 800-562-8088, www.physicianleaders.org

Essays 31 and 32: Adapted from an article originally published in *The Pharos*, Summer 2014, pages 34-37

Essay 33: https://www.kevinmd.com/2023/11/the-fine-line-between-childhood-illnesses-and-munchausen-syndrome-by-proxy.html

Essay 34

1. Michael Crichton quote: https://www.michaelcrichton.com/biography/doctor/

Essay 35:

1. "Company of One": https://www.kevinmd.com/2023/07/its-time-for-every-doctor-to-start-a-professional-micro-corporation.html#commentsModal

Essay 36

1. Simon D. Spivack quote: https://blogs.einsteinmed.edu/human-touch-an-essential-connection-between-patients-and-doctors

Essay 41

1. Aftermath of AHERF: https://www.proquest.com/docview/20006 5465?parentSessionId=jKSQknXUQLxbxTJ5swKXzhYI8pKVgnk EHAedm1XF%2FE4%3D&sourcetype=Scholarly%20Journals

Essay 42

1. Canadian Medical Education Journal: https://journalhosting.ucal-gary.ca/index.php/cmej/article/view/76086/56314

Essay 43

1. Jonathan A. Epstein, MD quote: https://www.inquirer.com/health/new-dean-perelman-school-of-medicine-20231213.html

Essay 44

1. Will Bunch quote: https://www.inquirer.com/columnists/at-tytood/gop-college-unc-chapel-hill-harvard-penn-dave-mccor-mick-20231219.html

2. Representative Elise Stefanik quote: https://stefanik.house. gov/2021/1/statement-congresswoman-stefanik-harvard-s-bowing-far-left

Essay 45

Harvard medical student essay: https://www.medpagetoday.com/opinion/second-opinions/107692

Milton Keynes UK
Ingram Content Group UK Ltd.
UKHW010641040324
438885UK00001B/205

9 798822 938984